CHILDHOOD DISORDERS
Behavioral-Developmental
Approaches

Other books from Banff International Conferences on Behavior Modification available from Brunner/Mazel

Behavior Modification and Families (Banff VI)
Behavior Modification Approaches to Parenting (Banff VI)
The Behavioral Management of Anxiety, Depression and Pain (Banff VII)
Behavioral Self-management: Strategies, Techniques and Outcome (Banff VIII)
Behavioral Systems for the Developmentally Disabled: I. School and Family Environments (Banff IX)
Behavioral Systems for the Developmentally Disabled: II. Institutional, Clinic and Community Environments (Banff IX)
Behavioral Medicine: Changing Health Lifestyles (Banff X)
Violent Behavior: Social Learning Approaches to Prediction, Management and Treatment (Banff XI)
Adherence, Compliance and Generalization in Behavioral Medicine (Banff XII)
Advances in Clinical Behavior Therapy (Banff XIV)

CHILDHOOD DISORDERS

Behavioral-Developmental

Approaches

Edited by

Robert J. McMahon

and

Ray DeV. Peters

BRUNNER/MAZEL, *Publishers* • New York

Library of Congress Cataloging in Publication Data

Banff International Conferences on Behavior Modification
(15th : 1983)
Childhood disorders.

Papers from the 15th of the Banff International
Conferences on Behavior Modification, held in 1983.
Includes bibliographies and indexes.
1. Child psychiatry—Congresses. 2. Behavioral
assessment of children—Congresses. 3. Child development
—Congresses. I. McMahon, Robert J. (Robert Joseph),
1953-   . II. Peters, Ray DeV., 1942-   . III. Title.
[DNLM: 1. Child Behavior Disorders—diagnosis—congresses.
2. Child Behavior Disorders—therapy—congresses. 3. Child
Development—congresses. W3 BA203 15th 1983c/
WS 350.6 B215 1983c]
RJ499.B26 1983   618.92'89   84-26341
ISBN 0-87630-379-3

Published by
Brunner/Mazel, Inc.
19 Union Square West
New York, New York 10003

Preface

This is one in a continuing series of publications sponsored by the Banff International Conferences on Behavioral Sciences. The conferences have been held each spring since 1969 in Banff, Alberta, Canada. They serve the purpose of bringing together outstanding behavioral scientists and professionals in a forum where they can present and discuss data related to emergent issues and topics. Thus, the International Conferences, as a continuing event, have served as an expressive "early indicator" of the developing nature and composition of behavioral science and scientific application.

Distance, schedules, and restricted audience preclude wide attendance at the conferences. Consequently, the publications have equal status with the conferences proper. They are not, however, simply publications of the papers presented at the conference. Major presenters at the Banff Conferences are required to write a chapter specifically for the forthcoming book, separate from their presentation and discussion at the conference itself.

The original conference had as its theme "Ideal Mental Health Services." The policy consciously adopted at that conference, and followed ever since, was to identify for the presentation of each year's theme those behavioral researchers who could best identify the state of the art. In 1969, the conference faculty were Nathan Azrin, Ogden Lindsley, Gerald Patterson, Todd Risley, and Richard Stuart.

The conference topics for the first five years were as follows:

1969: I.   IDEAL MENTAL HEALTH SERVICES
1970: II.   SERVICES AND PROGRAMS FOR EXCEPTIONAL CHILDREN AND YOUTH
1971: III. IMPLEMENTING BEHAVIORAL PROGRAMS FOR SCHOOLS AND CLINICS

1972: IV. BEHAVIOR CHANGE: METHODOLOGY, CONCEPTS, AND PRACTICE
1973: V.   EVALUATION OF BEHAVIORAL PROGRMS IN COMMUNITY, RESI-
           DENTIAL AND SCHOOL SETTINGS

Beginning in 1974, the Banff Conference books have been published by Brunner/Mazel, and the interested reader may obtain copies of these volumes from the publisher. (The proceedings of Banff XIII is not available.) The conference topics were:

1974: VI.   BEHAVIOR MODIFICATION AND FAMILIES and BEHAVIOR MODI-
            FICATION APPROACHES TO PARENTING
1975: VII. THE BEHAVIORAL MANAGEMENT OF ANXIETY, DEPRESSION AND
            PAIN
1976: VIII. BEHAVIORAL SELF-MANAGEMENT STRATEGIES, TECHNIQUES
            AND OUTCOMES
1977: IX.   BEHAVIORAL SYSTEMS FOR THE DEVELOPMENTALLY DISABLED:
            I. SCHOOL AND FAMILY ENVIRONMENTS
            II. INSTITUTIONAL, CLINIC, AND COMMUNITY ENVIRONMENTS
1978: X.   BEHAVIORAL MEDICINE: CHANGING HEALTH LIFESTYLES
1979: XI.   VIOLENT BEHAVIOR: SOCIAL LEARNING APPROACHES TO PRE-
            DICTION, MANAGEMENT AND TREATMENT
1980: XII. ADHERENCE, COMPLIANCE, AND GENERALIZATION IN BEHAV-
            IORAL MEDICINE
1981: XIII. ESSENTIALS OF BEHAVIORAL TREATMENTS FOR FAMILIES
1982: XIV. ADVANCES IN CLINICAL BEHAVIOR THERAPY

The Banff Conferences have been more than places where theories and research data are presented and discussed. The magnificence of the Banff natural environment and recreation opportunities, as well as the pleasurable ambience and resources of The Banff Centre where the conference is held, contribute enormously to the vigor and stimulation of the conference. It has encouraged substantial program development and evaluation and helped to bring together policymakers, program administrators, researchers, and clinicians in an effort to stimulate the adoption in practical settings of many of the programs that have been discussed during the conference proceedings.

The purpose of Banff XV was to focus on recent advances in the conceptualization, assessment, and treatment of childhood behavior disorders. While behavior disorders of children have been examined in several previous Banff Conferences, we wanted to pay particular attention to the role of developmental processes in the understanding and treatment of these disorders. To this end, invitations to participate in the Conference were extended to a group of clinicians who have incorporated developmental considerations to a significant degree in their research and applied work with children. This volume represents their contributions.

Over the years, many people have contributed notably to the success of these conferences. Those who have attended the conferences and participated so vigorously in the presentations and discussions, both formally and informally, contribute enormously to their success. In particular, we would also like to express our appreciation to Ms. Catherine Hardie and her staff in the Conferences Division at the Banff Centre. Catherine has been extensively involved in the planning and coordination of these conferences since 1973. Her outstanding organizational skills are matched only by her patience in dealing with a revolving committee of conference planners. In addition to the editors of this volume, other members of the conference Planning Committee who contributed substantial help and guidance to Banff XV were Dr. Kenneth D. Craig, Dr. L.A. Hamerlynck, and Dr. David E. Shearer.

Editing of this volume was supported in part by grants from the Social Sciences and Humanities Research Council of Canada and the National Institute of Mental Health.

R.J.M.
R. DeV. P.

Contents

Contributors

THOMAS M. ACHENBACH
University of Vermont

DONALD M. BAER
University of Kansas

RUSSELL A. BARKLEY
Medical College of Wisconsin

SALLY BARROS
University of Alberta

LINDA A. BREAM
University of Waterloo

DIANE BRICKER
University of Oregon

JAMES Y. CLARKE
*Mental Health Division
State of Oregon*

JANICE S. COHEN
University of Waterloo

NANCY C. GRIGG
University of Alberta

WILLIAM R. JENSON
*Children's Behavior Therapy
    Unit
Salt Lake County Mental Health
and
University of Utah*

MARILYN KANEE
University of Alberta

GERARD M. KYSELA
University of Alberta

DAVID LITTMAN
University of Oregon

SCOTT R. MCCONNELL
*Western Psychiatric Institute and
Clinic
University of Pittsburgh*

ROBERT J. MCMAHON
University of British Columbia

DONALD H. MEICHENBAUM
University of Waterloo

RAY DEV. PETERS
Queen's University

ARTHUR L. ROBIN
*Wayne State University School of
   Medicine*
and
Children's Hospital of Michigan

HILL M. WALKER
University of Oregon

DAVID A. WOLFE
University of Western Ontario

K. RICHARD YOUNG
Utah State University

Section I
CONCEPTUAL FOUNDATIONS

1

The Case for a Behavioral-Developmental Integrative Approach to the Assessment and Treatment of Childhood Disorders

ROBERT J. MCMAHON and
RAY DEV. PETERS

Clinical child psychology is the branch of clinical psychology concerned with the remediation of inappropriate patterns of behavior in children (Williams & Gordon, 1974). Although its theoretical foundations supposedly lie in both clinical and developmental psychology, the relevant research findings in the latter area have been largely ignored by clinicians. As a result, the two disciplines have often carried on research of mutual interest with little or no intercommunication.

It has only been within the past decade that clinicians have acknowledged the dearth of literature in clinical child psychology that utilizes developmental considerations, and have called for a rapprochement. Similarly, there has been a concomitant increase of interest among developmental psychologists in the contribution of developmental processes to the understanding of abnormal behavior in children. A good example of this emerging interest is the recent Special

Issue of *Child Development* (February, 1984) dedicated entirely to theoretical and empirical articles on developmental psychopathology.

While the potential for an integration of developmental and clinical child psychology seems enormous, there are relatively few studies that have employed such an approach. In general, there appear to be three areas of clinical child psychology in which developmental considerations can be viewed as potentially playing a major role. These include 1) models of psychopathology, 2) assessment and classification issues, and 3) the enhancement of treatment. In this introductory chapter, we will touch on some of the implications of an integration of behavioral-developmental approaches to these areas, and provide a brief overview of the chapters contained in this volume. These papers represent exemplars of the most recent theoretical and data-based attempts to integrate developmental findings into clinical child psychology.

MODELS OF PSYCHOPATHOLOGY

In 1974, Achenbach began the first edition of his text, *Developmental Psychopathology,* with the sentence, "This is a book about a field that hardly exists yet" (p. 3). In the second edition of the text, Achenbach (1982) noted that while there had been an increase in the amount of research related to the developmental aspects of psychopathology, much of the child psychopathology literature still continued to represent a downward extension of concepts, diagnoses, and methods borrowed from adult psychopathology.

The developmental approach to child psychopathology is aptly described in the observation that it should "help us to understand troublesome behavior in light of the developmental tasks, sequences, and processes that characterize human growth" (Achenbach, 1982, p. 1). According to Wenar (1982a, p. 201), there are two basic questions that must be dealt with in any model of developmental psychopathology: "What comprises normal development from infancy to adulthood?" and "What represents significant deviations from normal development?" The former question is, of course, the domain of developmental psychology, while the latter question is within the purview of clinical child psychology. Note, however, that answers to the second question are dependent upon a satisfactory resolution of the first.

At the most basic level, developmental considerations of child psychopathology have focused on the child's age (Campbell, 1983). While establishing which behaviors are problematic for children of different ages is a valuable first step, it is important to understand that chronological age and other demographic variables are merely marker variables. The underlying reasons for age differences in child behavior disorders may be due to a variety of factors. However, it remains for researchers to first document these developmental differences before subsequent research can be devoted to determining which variables are the bases for various developmental differences.

Regardless of whether we are charting the occurrence of child behavior disorders as a function of age, sex, or various cognitive variables such as intelligence or attributional style, we are still viewing the child at a single point in time. An important characteristic of developmental psychopathology is that the focus is on the "ontogenetic process whereby early patterns of individual adaptation evolve to later patterns of adaptation" (Sroufe & Rutter, 1984, p. 27). In other words, a true model of developmental psychopathology must move beyond a static conceptualization to one which views the child's behavior in the context of more long-term antecedents and consequences, i.e., in terms of etiology and prognosis (Wenar, 1982a). Wenar notes that the scarcity of developmental data concerning child psychopathology has mitigated against such an approach. In addition, he states that the popularity of behavioral approaches has also impeded the establishment of a truly developmental psychopathology, since behaviorists have focused on assessment and treatment rather than etiology or prognosis. However, the contents of this volume reflect the growing awareness of, and interest in, such developmental considerations by behavior therapists.

Developmental psychologists have stressed the likely complexity of the links between developmental processes and psychopathology (Sroufe & Rutter, 1984). Wenar (1982a) has described a number of "models" which may have heuristic value for examining these connections. In fixation, behavior that is appropriate at a certain age continues to be manifested at some later period in which it is no longer appropriate (e.g., thumbsucking in a 10-year-old). In regression, the child reverts to a behavior that he or she has outgrown. Another group of models includes behaviors that may be exaggerated, absent, or deficient compared to the behaviors of normal children. Qualitatively different behavior comprises another model of psychopathology. In this instance, Wenar is talking about behaviors that occur extremely rarely or only in unusual circumstances in the normal population, but which occur with a high degree of frequency in a disturbed child. Finally, there are the so-called developmental models, in which the child is assessed over time, so that patterns of development can be noted. Examples of this type of model include a slowed rate of growth compared to that of the general population, altered growth curves, an alteration in the variability of the growth curve, or one in which the sequencing of behaviors or stages of development is altered. Which, if any, of these models are applicable to a particular behavior or behavior disorder remains an empirical question.

ASSESSMENT

Developmental psychopathologists have stressed the necessity of defining psychopathology in the context of normal development (Achenbach, 1974, 1982; Garber, 1984; Wenar, 1982a, 1982b). In other words, these authors have recommended a normative comparison approach to psychopathology, and, by inference, to the processes of assessment and classification as well. Epidemiological studies have been the basis for most of the relevant information.

There has been a growing recognition of the utility of a developmental perspective in the field of child behavioral assessment (Edelbrock, 1984; Ollendick & Hersen, 1984). Edelbrock (1984) has described a "normative-developmental" approach to child behavioral assessment which stresses the utility of comparing children's behavior to a normative reference group (the "normative principle") and the necessity of considering the child's current level of functioning within the context of developmental antecedents and potential future consequences (the "developmental principle"). Specific operations of this approach include establishing normative baselines for behaviors of children of different ages, determining age differences in the patterning of child behaviors, and studying stability and changes in behaviors over time.

There are a number of advantages to utilizing normative comparisons in behavioral assessment (Hartmann, Roper, & Bradford, 1979). Such comparisons may permit a more precise formulation of the locus of the problem (e.g., child behavior versus parental perceptions of the behavior), assist in target behavior selection and evaluation of treatment outcome, and facilitate direct comparisons of research using different samples of children. However, there are a number of limitations as well (Campbell, 1983; Furman, 1980; Mash & Terdal, 1981). Typically, normative data on children's behavior has been based on global parental reports concerning the frequency of various child behaviors at different ages (Mash & Terdal, 1981). While global parent ratings of child behavior are an important source of data in child behavioral assessment (McMahon, 1984), they are subject to a variety of biasing factors. Frequency alone can be misleading as a sole indicator of deviance. Given that prevalence estimates for some single child behaviors may be very high at certain ages, it is important to take other dimensions of these behaviors into account (e.g., intensity, duration), as well as the relationship of a single behavior to other deviant behaviors (Garber, 1984). (Chapter 4 of this volume provides an exemplary demonstration of this latter approach.) In addition to normative comparisons based on parent report, direct observations of the child's behavior in a variety of situations are essential (Mash & Terdal, 1981). Finally, clinicians need to encourage the development and utilization of norms for prosocial behaviors as well.

In addition to the normative approach, there are at least two other approaches to behavioral assessment and, in particular, to the selection of the appropriate target behaviors for intervention, that include developmental considerations. These are a social validational approach and the "current and future adjustment" approach (Furman, 1980). Social validity refers to whether therapeutic changes are "socially or clinically important to the client" (Kazdin, 1977, p. 429). Developmental factors play a role in this assessment approach in that the perceived relevance of various child behaviors changes as a function of the child's developmental level, as do the actual behaviors themselves. For example, the development of children's interpersonal negotiation strategies with peers is a process that involves markedly different behaviors for children of different ages (Selman & Demorest, 1984).

In the current and future adjustment approach, target behaviors are selected for treatment on the basis of 1) whether they covary with a larger class of behaviors related to current adjustment, or 2) whether the behaviors are reliably associated with future difficulties. It is important to note that the specific predictors of current and future adjustment also change developmentally (Furman, 1980). This particular approach to behavioral assessment is quite consistent with the developmental psychopathology model.

TREATMENT

Clinicians, including behavior therapists, have been remiss in their failure to consider the relevance of developmental variables in treating child behavior disorders. For example, a review of the contents of two influential behavioral journals, *Behavior Therapy* and the *Journal of Applied Behavior Analysis,* failed to locate a single study which examined the relative effectiveness of a behavioral intervention with children of different ages (Furman, 1980). Less than 25% of a sample of the articles from these journals even mentioned developmental factors.

In a seminal contribution, Furman (1980) described a variety of developmental implications for the enhancement of social development in children. In addition to the developmental concerns regarding target behavior selection discussed above, he has also documented the significance of developmental factors in the application of traditional behavioral techniques and the development of new interventions for improving the social competency of children. For example, with respect to social reinforcement, younger children are more responsive to social praise while older children are more responsive to accuracy feedback (e.g., "right") (Lewis, Wall, & Aronfreed, 1963). Preschool children of both sexes are more responsive to praise from adult females, while older children are more responsive to praise from an opposite sex adult (Stevenson, 1965). When compared with social praise, material rewards decrease in incentive value with increasing age (Witryol, 1971). Symbolic rewards appear to increase in incentive value with age as compared to material rewards (Harter, 1975). With respect to the development of new intervention procedures, Furman briefly describes the developmental literature concerning rules, rationales, and social cognitive skills. This paper is required reading for those clinicians and clinical researchers interested in the applicability of developmental variables to clinical treatment methods.

Other behavior therapists have acknowledged the potential relevance of developmental considerations to child behavior therapy. Harris and Ferrari (1983) recently reviewed the literature concerning attention deficit disorder and children's fears, and suggested ways in which developmental factors might be incorporated into behavioral interventions for these disorders. Cognitive-behavioral therapists have also called for increased consideration of developmental factors (e.g., Kendall, Lerner, & Craighead, 1984). For example, Copeland (1981, 1982) discussed a variety of subject variables that should be recognized and assessed in evaluating the effectiveness of cognitive self-instruction and other self-management procedures. Harter (1982) has provided an excellent discussion of her work on the role of developmental processes in both internal and external reward systems.

In our own research endeavors, we have also attempted to incorporate developmental considerations into intervention procedures. McMahon and his colleagues at the University of British Columbia have conducted a series of laboratory studies with nonreferred ("normal") children examining whether various behavioral parenting skills (ignoring, time out, positive reinforcement) are differentially effective with children of different ages (three to four-and-a-half versus five-and-a-half to seven-and-a-half), and whether including a verbal rationale or a rationale plus modeling procedure for the child enhances the effects of these various parenting skills. In the study of ignoring, Davies, McMahon, Flessati, and Tiedemann (1984) found that having mothers provide a verbal rationale and/or model an ignoring procedure for the child prior to its use enhanced child compliance to maternal commands, reduced the extinction burst phenomenon associated with ignoring, and enhanced parental satisfaction with the ignoring procedure. The procedures were equally effective with children of different ages, although the older children were more compliant than the younger children. Both of the adjunctive procedures (rationale and rationale plus modeling) were equally effective. In the second investigation (McMahon, Davies, & Tiedemann, 1983), time out was the behavioral parenting technique of focus. While the adjunctive procedures did not enhance child compliance to maternal commands over the time-out procedure alone, the adjuncts did facilitate a reduction in inappropriate child behaviors such as whining, crying, aggression, and smart talk. Data from the positive reinforcement study are currently being analyzed.

Thus, the potential value of integrating developmental processes with assessment and treatment procedures and models of childhood disorders appears to be substantial, even though the attempts to do so have only recently begun. The major purpose of the present volume is to provide examples of how developmental considerations are currently being incorporated into the analysis and treatment of various behavior problems in children.

OVERVIEW OF THE VOLUME

This volume is divided into two major sections. In the first three chapters (including this chapter), we have attempted to provide the reader with an overview of the conceptual foundations of a behavioral-developmental approach to child behavior disorders. The next two chapters in this section describe the applied behavior-analytic and cognitive-behavioral approaches, respectively.

Applied behavior analysis has established itself as an effective approach for dealing with a wide variety of childhood disorders. One of its most eloquent spokesmen, Don Baer, presents the case for perceiving applied behavior analysis as a "conceptually conservative" view of childhood disorders. It is conservative in that the term "behavior disorder" is seen as a concept arising from the complaints of others about certain child behaviors, and therefore includes in its analysis the behavior of the complainants. It is also conservative in the sense that the concept of cause is not viewed as necessary to the successful remediation of maladaptive behavior. Baer presents a strong logical argument supporting the view that child behavior is subject to the same laws of behavior as during any other period of the lifespan.

Meichenbaum, Bream, and Cohen present the basic tenets of the cognitive-behavioral perspective of child behavior disorders. Given the emphasis on cognitive processes in this approach, the literature on children's cognitive development assumes paramount importance in the construction and selection of appropriate assessment and intervention procedures for children. Meichenbaum and his colleagues use the example of the socially withdrawn child to explicate the role of the cognitive-behavioral perspective with respect to child behavior disorders. They review the developmental literature concerning peer relationships and offer clear suggestions as to how these data can be integrated into the assessment and subsequent treatment of the socially withdrawn child.

In the second section of the book, we present a variety of examples of successful models and programs for the assessment and treatment of various childhood disorders from infancy through adolescence. While these chapters describe a variety of assessment and treatment methods with different populations of children, the common thread is that they have all incorporated developmental considerations to a significant degree.

Achenbach provides a powerful argument for the utilization of taxometric systems in the diagnosis and assessment of child behavior disorders. Following a brief review of the strengths and weaknesses of behavioral assessment, clinically derived classification systems such as the DSM-III and earlier multivariate approaches, he describes a taxometric approach to diagnosis and assessment. Taxometry can increase our understanding of child behavior disorders by allowing us to aggregate molecular assessment data into more molar units, by providing a normative-developmental context in which to judge the behavior of particular children, and by facilitating the grouping of children according to overall patterns of behavior in order to establish profile types. Achenbach illustrates this approach by describing his own research with the Child Behavior Checklist and the Child Behavior Profile.

Early intervention models of treatment for handicapped or at-risk infants have become established as viable intervention strategies (Tjossem, 1976). A basic requirement for the implementation of such a program is an assessment device that reliably discriminates those infants who are developing normally from those who are not. Bricker and Littman point out that such a detection system must be able to accurately identify at-risk infants, and it must not be prohibitively expensive. They describe their work in the development of a long-term monitoring system for at-risk infants using the parents as monitors of their infant's development.

The next two chapters describe models for the integration of handicapped children into the regular school setting. In both chapters, the literature on the controversial issue of "mainstreaming" handicapped children into less restrictive settings such as the regular classroom is reviewed. Kysela and his colleagues then describe their decision-making model for integration into preschool settings. The model depends on information regarding the child and his or her family; synthesis of these data into a program for the child; implementation of the program utilizing classroom personnel, peers, and family members; and ongoing program review and modification. Developmental processes of the child are considered at all stages of the model. As Kysela and his colleagues note, the model awaits empirical evaluation. Nonetheless, it is a notable example of systematic planning for integration of the handicapped child and will likely facilitate refinements to this often difficult process.

Walker, McConnell, and Clarke describe the development of a program designed to facilitate the social integration of handicapped elementary school-aged children into less restrictive settings. The SBS (Social Behavior Survival) model provides handicapped children with the behavioral skills and competencies necessary for successful adjustment in the classroom, both in terms of the teachers' expectations and with respect to the nonhandicapped peer group as well. The SBS program contains both assessment and intervention components, and preliminary evaluations of both components indicate the potential value of this model. Normative data on the SBS assessment devices are also being collected.

One of the most serious childhood disorders is infantile autism. It is also one of the most mystifying. Jenson and Young draw on their considerable expertise in working with this population of children to describe the developmental and behavioral characteristics of autism, the prognosis for these children at later stages of development, and the behavioral interventions that have proven effective in treatment. The core behavior management programs developed by Jenson, and Young's success in employing nonhandicapped peer tutors with autistic children, are exciting innovations in helping these children.

Wolfe then discusses his work in the prevention of child abuse by promoting the development of competency in both the parent and child. The goals of such a program include parental acquisition of more effective parenting strategies early in the child's life, improved coping mechanisms for the parent, and development of child adaptive behaviors that will facilitate his or her adjustment. Wolfe identifies a number of parental and child risk factors based on the child abuse and developmental literatures, and provides examples of how such risk factors are being modified in his own work with these high-risk families.

In the next chapter, Barkley describes the results of his programmatic research on the social behavior of hyperactive children. He focuses on parent-child interactions in particular, and discusses the differential effects that types of interaction (free play versus task completion), age of the child, and medication dosage have on parent and child interactional behaviors. The studies suggest, among other things, that hyperactive children may suffer a lag in the development of compliance and self-control relative to their normal peers, and that negative maternal behavior toward the hyperactive child may be a *result* of the child's behavior as opposed to a causal factor.

Robin then reviews the developmental characteristics of families in which there is an adolescent child. He describes a behavioral-family systems model to account for parent-adolescent conflict, and an intervention program to restore the family to a more adaptive level of functioning. Robin's research on the effectiveness of the Problem-Solving Communication Training program is also described. The findings suggest that this approach to dealing with parent-adolescent conflict is a useful one.

CONCLUSION

It is apparent that there is increased recognition among both developmental and clinical child psychologists of the potential utility of adopting an integrative approach to conceptualizing, assessing, and treating child behavior disorders. Clinical child psychologists, including those employing behavioral and social learning approaches, have much to gain from this collaborative endeavor. It is our hope that the ideas and research discussed in this volume will encourage and facilitate communication among clinical and developmental psychologists in the search for a better understanding, as well as more effective treatment, of childhood behavior disorders.

REFERENCES

ACHENBACH, T. M. (1974). *Developmental psychopathology* (1st edition). New York: Ronald Press.

ACHENBACH, T. M. (1982). *Developmental psychopathology* (2nd edition). New York: Wiley.

CAMPBELL, S. B. (1983). Developmental perspectives in child psychopathology. In T. H. Ollendick & M. Hersen (Eds.), *Handbook of child psychopathology* (pp. 13-40). New York: Plenum.

COPELAND, A. P. (1981). The relevance of subject variables in cognitive self-instructional programs for impulsive children. *Behavior Therapy, 12*, 520-529.

COPELAND, A. P. (1982). Individual difference factors in children's self-management: Toward individualized treatments. In P. Karoly & F. H. Kanfer (Eds.), *Self-management and behavior change: From theory to practice* (pp. 207-239). New York: Pergamon.

DAVIES, G. R., McMAHON, R. J., FLESSATI, E. W., & TIEDEMANN. G. L. (1984). Verbal rationales and modeling as adjuncts to a parenting technique for child compliance. *Child Development, 55*, 1290-1298.

EDELBROCK, C. (1984). Developmental considerations. In. T. H. Ollendick & M. Hersen (Eds.), *Child behavioral assessment: Principles and procedures* (pp. 20-37). New York: Pergamon.

FURMAN, W. (1980). Promoting social development: Developmental implications for treatment. In B. B. Lahey & A. E. Kazdin (Eds.), *Advances in clinical child psychology* (Vol. 3, pp. 1-40). New York: Plenum.

GARBER, J. (1984). Classification of childhood psychopathology: A developmental perspective. *Child Development, 55*, 30-48.

HARRIS, S. L., & FERRARI. M. (1983). Developmental factors in child behavior therapy. *Behavior Therapy, 14*, 54-72.

HARTER, S. (1975). Developmental differences in the manifestation of mastery motivation on problem-solving tasks. *Child Development, 46*, 370-378.

HARTER, S. (1982). A developmental perspective on some parameters of self-regulation in children. In P. Karoly & F. H. Kanfer (Eds.), *Self-management and behavior change: From theory to practice* (pp. 165-204). New York: Pergamon.

HARTMANN, D. P., ROPER, B. L., & BRADFORD, D. C. (1979). Some relationships between behavioral and traditional assessment. *Journal of Behavioral Assessment, 1,* 3-21.

KAZDIN, A. E. (1977). Assessing the clinical or applied importance of behavior change through social validation. *Behavior Modification, 1,* 427-452.

KENDALL, P. C., LERNER, R. M., & CRAIGHEAD, W. E. (1984). Human development and intervention in childhood psychopathology. *Child Development, 55,* 71-82.

LEWIS, M., WALL, A. M., & ARONFREED, J. (1963). Developmental change in the relative values of social and non-social reinforcement. *Journal of Experimental Psychology, 66,* 133-137.

MASH, E. J., & TERDAL, L. G. (1981). Behavioral assessment of childhood disturbance. In E. J. Mash & L. G. Terdal (Eds.), *Behavioral assessment of childhood disorders* (pp. 3-76). New York: Guilford.

MCMAHON, R. J. (1984). Behavioral checklists and rating forms. In T. H. Ollendick & M. Hersen (Eds.), *Child behavioral assessment: Principles and procedures* (pp. 80-105). New York: Pergamon.

MCMAHON, R. J., DAVIES, G. R., & TIEDEMANN, G. L. (1983, December). *Developmental considerations in using time out: Adjunctive procedures and age effects.* Paper presented at the World Congress on Behavior Therapy, Washington, DC.

OLLENDICK, T. H., & HERSEN, M. (1984). An overview of child behavioral assessment. In T. H. Ollendick & M. Hersen (Eds.), *Child behavioral assessment: Principles and procedures* (pp. 3-19). New York: Pergamon.

SELMAN. R. L., & DEMOREST, A. P. (1984). Observing troubled children's interpersonal negotiation strategies: Implications of and for a developmental model. *Child Development, 55,* 288-304.

SROUFE, L. A., & RUTTER, M. (1984). The domain of developmental psychopathology. *Child Development, 55,* 17-29.

STEVENSON, H. W. (1965). Social reinforcement of children's behavior. In L. P. Lipsett & C. C. Spiker (Eds.), *Advances in child development and behavior* (Vol. 2, pp. 97-126). New York: Academic Press.

TJOSSEM, T. D. (Ed.). (1976). *Intervention strategies for high-risk infants and young children.* Baltimore: University Park Press.

WENAR, C. (1982a). Developmental psychopathology: Its nature and models. *Journal of Clinical Child Psychology, 11,* 192-201.

WENAR, C. (1982b). *Psychopathology from infancy through adolescence: A developmental approach.* New York: Random House.

WILLIAMS, G. J., & GORDON, S. (Eds.). (1974). *Clinical child psychology: Current practices and future perspectives.* New York: Behavioral Publications.

WITRYOL, S. L. (1971). Incentives and learning in children. In H. W. Reese (Ed.), *Advances in child development and behavior* (Vol. 6, pp. 1-61). New York: Academic Press.

2

Applied Behavior Analysis as a Conceptually Conservative View of Childhood Disorders

DONALD M. BAER

There is an analytic view of behavior called behavior analysis. As a result, there is a behavior-analytic view of any aspect of the universe in which the behavior of an organism can figure. To say that something is an aspect of the universe means that we can distinguish it in some way from the other aspects of the universe. Interestingly, applying a behavior-analytic view to an aspect of the universe sometimes shows that we no longer need to view it any other way—it no longer needs separation, at least not from those other parts of the universe in which the behavior of organisms is central. In particular, a behavior-analytic view of childhood suggests that when the behavior of children is analyzed, childhood is not a separate collection of phenomena, in that it has few if any principles unique to itself: It connects to the rest of the universe of behavior so thoroughly that it gains nothing from being segregated as if its connections were primarily internal—indeed, it loses something fundamental to its best and most general analysis.

However, people behave about children as if children were a distinctively important state of the organism. This has not often been true

17

in history, but it is true now in some parts of the world, and so, to that extent, childhood becomes a behavioral phenomenon—not in itself, but in the way that people relate to it.

How people behave about children is itself subject to behavioral analysis, of course. When it is analyzed, it too disappears as an aspect worthy of categorization, because its principles and relationships are seen as better connected to the universe of behavior as such than to some smaller domain called *relating to children*. Even so, blissfully ignorant of that analysis, many people continue to behave toward children as if children were a distinctive phenomenon of life. Thus, we create roles for children, build institutions for them, dictate their curricula within and outside those institutions, define part of our economy in terms of them, and encourage them to define a subculture of their own which we then cheerfully sell to them even as we bemoan much of it. In general, we take responsibility for our children to such an extent that subsequent letting go of it can become one of the crises of our joint lives.

We do all that, obedient of course to the principles of behavior in general rather than to some specialized principles of behavior about children and about relating to them; and in the process of doing so, we define disorders of childhood. These truly are disorders that we define, for in no sense are the children disorderly. The children are simply doing what the principles of behavior require them to do; it is we who have constructed a larger environment around them such that some of the things that children naturally do will not fit comfortably into that environment. Often, the discomfort is more ours than the children's; sometimes, it is theirs, too—we take care to share it with them.

Thus, we rear children in small social units called families, and create a culture that expects the children to be thoroughly under social control, and only social control, within their families. But we do not teach family adults the principles and tactics of social control—indeed, we have not known the principles very long, and the tactics are still being developed. When the children are not brought under enough social control by these amateurs, we call the children oppositional, emotionally disturbed, schizophrenic, and autistic, for a start. When the adults exhaust the meagre supply of tactics that they have learned from the examples of their parents, their neighbors, and their cultural media, they sometimes fall back on the physically coercive tactics that work so well with the material objects and devices of their environment; we call these parents abusive and their children abused. In any event, we send the children to school for many years, and design the school to operate under much the same social control that we thought the family was using successfully. We present them with a curriculum to learn, on the assumption that it progresses in easy enough steps so that any child can learn it all in the sequence in which it is offered. Most of us, after all, learned some of it in that sequence. When children prove not to be under instructional control in school, we continue to call them oppositional, disturbed, schizophrenic, and autistic for a start; when the school, like the parents, naturally devolves into aversive techniques of control and the children develop avoidance behaviors, we call them school-phobic and a number of other DSM titles, as well. When the children seem to be under reasonable social control—or at least are not disruptive—yet fail to learn the curriculum in the order in which we assign it, we call them unintelligent, retarded, and if they are selective in what they fail to learn, learning-disabled.

All of these deviant responses we consider childhood disorders, but the disorders are in the match between the environments that we arrange for our children and the behaviors that we expect them to develop in those environments. According to a behavior-analytic view the children are very orderly in their response to all these environments; they are doing what they must. So are we: We arrange their environments as best we know, and in obedience to the forces in our own environments, some of which are the normative behavior patterns of our children. There is no blame in this view of us, only interdependency.

Just as there is no blame, there is no pathology. A behavior-analytic view of behavior understands all behavior in terms of its controlling functions. It categorizes behavior according to what function it serves, and it categorizes functions according to the form of behavior change that they accomplish and the procedures that embody them. Thus, behaviors are classified according to whether their control is by antecedent or consequent stimuli in their environments; and functions are classified according to whether they use antecedents or consequences, and whether they increase behavior, decrease it, or set it into a known pattern of relationship with other stimuli, other behaviors, and time. Nowhere in these classifications is there a concept of good or bad behavior, healthy or pathological, ordered or disordered. The concept of a behavior disorder is not in our science of behavior analysis, but in our behavior: We *complain* about some of our children's behaviors.

This point is worth emphasizing to this extent because if we are to intervene—and probably we are—we should remember that the complaint is as subject to behavioral analysis as is the behavior being complained about. And if neither is a disorder, we have a choice: Shall we modify the behavior complained about, or modify the complaining behavior? The premise that neither is pathological suggests that a conservative approach to the problem will question first the behavior of complaining. After all, the children are doing what they should be doing, not in our terms, perhaps, but in their environment's terms, certainly. If that does not suit us, then whose problem is it? Ours—at least at first glance.

Second glance suggests less clarity in this priority, of course. Granted, the children are doing just what they should be doing in response to their environment; but so are the complainers. Furthermore, the complainers are adult, often numerous, and occasionally assumed to represent not merely individuals but us, sometimes called Society. Even when they don't, they are bigger, stronger, richer, and a lot more in charge than the children. We have a long baseline of deciding that even if the children are doing what their environment requires, when we do what our environment requires and that turns out to be not liking what the children do, *we* change *their* behavior, first labeling it in a manner that will justify our intervention. We also point out that we can foresee the long-term consequences of the children continuing to behave in their current undesirable manner, and that they are bad consequences; we usually do not point out that we arranged those future situations that the children's behavior won't fit well, and that rather than change our long-term arrangements, we shall change their current behavior disorder, or at least segregate it more or less out of our way.

Again, there is no blame in this situation, if behavior analysis is correct in its assumptions; there is only a set of interactions responsive to their current and past environments, in which we see the possibility of intervention. Seeing them as interactions may clarify seeing some paths of intervention; seeing them behavior-analytically may allow us to see rather more interventions (like those aimed at the complainer), and to see them pragmatically, in terms of everybody's environmental presses, rather than moralistically, in terms of who's disordered and who isn't. Imposing a value of order, or health, or developmental integrity complicates these interactions well beyond what their analysis as behavioral interactions requires. Thus, the behavior-analytic view of them is conservative compared to the developmental or pathology-oriented point of view. Furthermore, if imposing a value of order, health, or developmental propriety on children's behavior is seen as just one more behavioral interaction of the adults who do it, then it simply invites analysis, not belief; but if that value is seen as *correctly* imposed, then it invites belief and thus requires proof rather than analysis. That proof will be extraordinarily demanding and difficult to assemble. Needing it is thus the opposite of conservative; defensible, of course, but far from conservative. Reckless, one might say.

None of this argument denies the possibility that there is indeed a standard of healthy, developmentally proper child behavior. The argument only points out that: 1) such a proposition does not appear in a behavior-analytic view of child behavior; 2) asserting that it is nevertheless correct is a behavior capable of behavior analysis to demonstrate the conditions under which people assert it or do not; 3) asserting that it is nevertheless correct imposes an obligation of proof apart from analysis of the conditions under which people assert that it is correct; and 4) the proof will be very lengthy and difficult, perhaps because the assertion is wrong.

In medicine, the situation is sometimes simpler. Some physiological, biochemical processes of the organism, while just as natural as others, nevertheless bring the organism to death; these can easily be called pathological. But the moment that we observe that some behaviors, while just as natural as others, nevertheless bring their organism to death, we remember that sometimes these behaviors are considered self-sacrifice, unselfish, moral, and developmentally very advanced, at least when they serve certain social functions loosely labeled heroism or righteousness. Absent that social function, they are loosely termed self-destructive behavior and routinely subjected to intervention—yet in some cultures, a child doing that might well be simply practicing for future heroism or, at least, survival in the face of physical adversity, and praise rather than therapy would be applied. In our culture, a child doing that might be seeking the attention of certain adults who cannot tolerate letting it continue; or guaranteeing the inattention of the adults who cannot tolerate their inability to deal with it; or making something happen in an environment in which he or she does not know how to make anything else happen; or is responding to an internal biochemical process that either elicits this behavior despite its consequences, or somehow makes these consequences reinforcing.

The point is that every one of these processes has been seen or suspected to operate at various times in various children. When we see self-destructive behavior, we do not know instantly that we are looking at pathology. We need analysis of this behavior before we can categorize it, and only one of the analyses just listed—the biochemical process—looks pathological.* The other potential analyses once again represent not pathology but a mismatch between the inevitable results of the child's environment and our expectations of what should happen in that environment, and our limited knowledge of how to have made a better environment in which the child's behavior would match our expectations.

Does the child's self-injurious behavior serve an attention-seeking function? That can happen—but only because it does not suit us and our arrangements to give the child a properly trained adult. Properly trained adults know how to avoid such traps, and can teach children to seek their attention by more acceptable behavior. Furthermore, they can establish their approval as a positive reinforcer, their disapproval as a negative reinforcer and punisher, and their attention as neither. Such adults are expensive to train; this analysis is tantamount to saying that it does not suit our knowledge, our beliefs, and our arrangements of the world to pay that much for the care of children likely to become self-injurious. But the key point is that the analysis centers finally on what controls what we know, believe, and will spend our money on, and not on a concept of healthy behavior.

Does the child's self-injurious behavior serve an attention-avoiding function? That too can happen—but only because it again did not suit us and our arrangements to give the child a properly trained adult. Properly trained adults know how to mediate more positive than negative outcomes of their interactions with the child. Granted, adults must make demands on the child throughout the day; even so, it is possible to do that in ways that bring the child to reinforcement rather than punishment—it is simply a matter of the adults' skill. Again, such adults are expensive to train; again, the source of the child's problem is not pathology in the child, but those contingencies in our world that govern what we know, believe, and will spend on the education and training of the adults who care for children, whether they are the child's parents or an institution's staff.

Does the child's self-injurious behavior serve a self-stimulatory function, in an environment in which the child does not know how to make anything else stimulating happen? If so, that can only be because it did not suit us and our arrangements to give the child a properly

---

* But even in that case, we should first be sure that this is indeed a biochemical process, not a matter of social or ecological contingencies; and even if that becomes clear, we should then ask about the antecedents of that biochemical process: Is it possible that they are social or ecological?

trained adult whose expertise includes knowing how to teach a child to exploit the ecological contingencies in the child's environment. Granted, the adult cannot provide well-designed social contingencies all day; even so, it is possible to enrich the ecology of even a profoundly retarded child's environment enough to occupy the isolate child's behavior; doing so means that we are willing to buy the equipment necessary for such an environment, and train adults to introduce children effectively to that equipment. Behavior-analytically, that is the source of the child's problem, and none of that is pathological; it is merely unattractive to acknowledge for what it is.

These arguments may not remind us of what we usually mean by the term *conservative*. Politically, they probably sound radical rather than conservative. As Skinner (1974) points out in explaining the term *radical behaviorism,* the dictionary's first meaning of *radical* is basic, profound, fundamental, or at the root or going to the source of something; its second meaning is favoring *fundamental* change. These arguments have, in the paradigm of behavior analysis, gone to the source of the problems that they cite, as behavior-analytic logic recognizes sources; and each time the source turns out to be the behavior of someone, then behavior-analytic logic can continue to ask for a behavioral analysis of *their* behavior. The analysis, of course, always will look to environmental causes; as soon as those causes stop turning out to be someone's behavior, analysis can stop, content with a meaningful answer—in its terms of what constitutes meaning.

Then we have the agreeable spectacle of an analysis being a radically conservative analysis. It is conservative in that it does not add an extremely problematic concept of disorder to the analysis of behavior, already empirically well begun without such a concept; and it is radical in that it postulates the environment as pragmatically the fundamental cause of the behaviors that invite the imprudent use of the term *behavior disorder*.

But did it truly postulate the fundamental causes of those behaviors? The form of the argument seemed satisfactory, behavior-analytically. What if it were argued from a different, non-behavior-analytic standpoint, though? In other words, what are the conditions that govern how curious, analytic people use a term like *fundamental cause?* Which is to say, what is the behavioral analysis of postulating fundamental causes? I have tried tackling that problem before (Deitz & Baer, 1982); let me try it again here.

I will begin with a homely example. A colleague in a different department of my university routinely asks me every year to lecture—once—to her introductory experimental psychology class. Nominally, I have one function there, which is to illustrate single-subject designs, so that her students will know that these designs exist and have certain uses. I suspect that I also serve two other functions, albeit implicitly: one is to portray the probability that these designs are not worth more than one hour with someone who does not contribute questions to the exams, and another is to show that she is very broad-minded, as indeed she is.

On one of these richly symbolic occasions, I had used as an example a reversal design showing that a preschool child's peer-interaction rate could be controlled by teachers' social reinforcement of certain easy-to-recognize members of that response class. I chose the example deliberately, supposing that my colleague's criticism of it would focus on its apparent lack of generality across children. I would then remark that the students in our undergraduate and Master's level early-education programs had done that problem (as a training exercise) about 100 times in the last 15 years, almost always with similar results, and that was the way that generality ought to be examined. Instead, she asserted that the study was a convincing example of how you could *control* a child's peer-interaction rate, but had not established the *cause* of the child's initial low peer-interaction rate. Would I claim that the child had entered preschool "shy" because of a lack of contingent adult attention? That, she said with emphatic finality, would be like claiming that the cause of a headache was an absence of aspirin. Fortunately for me, that class ended at just that moment, and so her students left without discovering that I did not have an articulate answer coming from a stimulus-control analysis of what we mean by "cause"; fortunately for her, she had to leave immediately for her next class elsewhere, and so did not discover that neither did she, for my tactic would have been to ask her for one. Since she is not available for an analysis of the stimulus controls of her usage of that word, let us consider our own cases.

Are any of you uncomfortable with the assertion that a cause of headache is an absence of aspirin? I was, but I'm not anymore. Why not? Perhaps I can approach the answer with a parallel question: Are you uncomfortable with the assertion that a cause of scurvy is an absence of vitamin C in the diet? I'm not, and never was, probably in part because of my extreme ignorance of biochemistry. However, the biochemists whom I know are also quite comfortable with the assertion that an absence of vitamin C is a cause of scurvy, and quite uncomfortable with the assertion that an absence of aspirin is a cause of headache. Yet within moments of considering this quandary, they suggest the case of the guinea pig that does not synthesize vitamin C in itself and so is totally dependent on external—typically, dietary—sources; in the absence of such sources, it is tiny, shriveled, weak, and quick to die. I know a few people who take aspirin constantly to remain free of headache or arthritic pain or muscular pain; and I know of guinea pigs who eat vitamin-C foods constantly to remain alive. Why should we be comfortable with the assertion of cause in the vitamin-C case but not in the aspirin case?

Perhaps *apparent universality* is one answer: All guinea pigs are alike in their requirement for vitamin C if they are to avoid scurvy, yet very few humans require constant aspirin ingestion to remain generally free of headaches and other pains. Any guinea pig, then, will show clear responsiveness to an ABABAB . . . reversal design, in which A is the absence of vitamin C and B is its adequate presence; only a few humans will show similar experimental control in a design in which A is the absence of aspirin and B is its adequate presence. Most humans will report near-zero levels of long-term pain in the *absence* of aspirin—then how can an absence of aspirin be a cause of pain, for them? The key term in that observation was "near-zero levels of long-term pain" in the absence of aspirin. In the presence of aspirin, those same humans probably will report even-nearer-to-zero levels of long-term pain than in its absence. An experimental design extending over very long periods of time, and using rather large time intervals within which to quantify presence or absence of long-term pain, after all may look very responsive to an ABABAB . . . reversal design in which A is the absence of aspirin and B is its adequate presence.

All that I have done here is adjust two temporal parameters, and apparent universality suddenly emerges as clearly across humans and their aspirin-remediable pains as it does across guinea pigs and their vitamin C-remediable scurvy. Surely our usages of a term like *cause* do not depend on merely the adjustment of a few temporal parameters—or do they? If they do, and if any of us is uncomfortable with the value of applied behavior analysis as being technological rather than scientific, then we may have discovered some of the stimulus controls that account for our use of those labels, and thus for our discomfort. If so, then a superordinate question presents itself, perhaps an essentially behavior-therapeutic question: Is a mere adjustment in a few temporal parameters worth that much discomfort, or should we try for a new organization of this aspect of our behavior?

Perhaps *apparent priority* is another answer to when we are comfortable invoking "cause" and when we aren't: Headache appears first, and aspirin then remediates it; a child arrives at preschool already shy, and contingent teacher attention then creates high rates of peer interaction. But take vitamin C out of the diet, and then scurvy appears in consequence. Thus, we can ask about the "causes" of the headache apart from the aspirin that subsequently remediated it after it had appeared, and we can ask about the "causes" of the child's shyness apart from the contingent teacher attention that remediated it after it had appeared; but we tend not to ask about the "causes" of scurvy apart from a vitamin-C deficiency, and so we may think that there are no causes of it apart from the vitamin-C deficiency. But what is scurvy? It is at least a thoroughgoing inadequacy and disintegration of connective tissue throughout the organism, and it is a disruption in oxidation processes, especially at the membranes of the blood cells; thus it is a syndrome of anemia, weakness, easy bleeding from the mucous membranes, spongy gums and frequent loss of teeth, and premature death. Is the absence of vitamin C the only cause of these effects? Certainly not; each of them can be made to happen through some variety of mechanisms. Vitamin C happens to participate crucially in some of the mechanisms controlling each of these effects, but not in all of them.

Thus, scurvy is a disease only in that it is the concatenation of anemia, weakness, and disintegration of connective tissue all at the same time: Its components all can be caused not only by vitamin-C deficiency but by other events as well. If those other events happen to be arranged in a suitable concatenation, then all of these effects would result, and we would look at them and perhaps say scurvy, but vitamin-C deficiency would not be the cause this time. The components of scurvy, after all, are like headache and shyness, in that they too are subject to multiple causation. Any effects that are subject to multiple causation can thus precede the particular cause that we apply to them when we control them; and so, when we control them, we are dealing with *a* cause, not *the* cause. Any time that we are dealing with *a* cause, not *the* cause, we are likely to find the problem, the effect, or the phenomenon already in existence prior to our management of it with our choice from among its several causes. That does not make our cause any less a cause; it only makes it clear that our cause is *a* cause and not *the* cause. Probably, in any aspect of the natural world, it will be rare to deal with phenomena that have one cause rather than many. Are any of us still uncomfortable with the assertion that an absence of aspirin is *a* cause of headache, and an absence of teacher attention contingent on peer interaction is *a* cause of a child's shyness? Could that discomfort be under the unrecognized stimulus control of search for *the* cause rather than *a* cause? If so, then again a superordinate behavior-therapeutic question arises: Is that stimulus control worth complicating the field, or would we consider shifting that stimulus control from an intraverbal *the* to an intraverbal *a*?

Perhaps multiple causation causes some of us no discomfort, in that we know that headaches, peer interaction, and scurvy have multiple causes, always did, and always will. The problem is that we are reinforced by knowing the specific immediate cause of the effect that we are studying, the one cause of the many possible that in fact happens to be responsible this time. Thus, we already know that headaches can result from a variety of ion misbalances, vascular conditions, muscular strains, and aspirin absences, and we suspect that they can result from some other factors as well that no one has yet analyzed. But Client 3 happens to have a headache right now, and we want to discover which of those known and unknown causes is *the* cause of *this* headache. I can think of two reasons why we would want to know that: 1) to see if the cause of this headache is one of the familiar, already analyzed causes, which discovery will contribute a mite to the generality of that analysis; or to see if it is not, and instead represents some new mechanism of headache production, which, if we can clarify it, might considerably enrich our understanding of headaches, and perhaps of pain in general, and perhaps of behavior in general, which is a superb reason; or 2) because that's what turns us on.

The first case represents a standard instance of scientific curiosity, the results of which are always valuable to the field. In either case, though, the problem is to discern the research tactics necessary to discovering what *the* cause of *this* specific headache is. The only tactic that I know, so far, is to manipulate some variable experimentally to see if it alleviates or intensifies this headache. But that tactic would show that aspirin administration is exactly such a variable. A complementary ecological examination of Client 3's recent history might well show that Client 3 had not had aspirin for some time, and so I might conclude that aspirin absence could be a cause of Client 3's headache. Still, I would be unable to assert that it was *the* cause of Client 3's headache.

In the same way, I might show that Client 3 was muscularly tense, and that the administration of systematic-relaxation instructions could alleviate the headache; again, ecological examination of Client 3's recent history might well show a recent absence of systematic-relaxation instructions or performance. So I might conclude that the absence of systematic-relaxation instructions or performance could be a cause of this headache. Still, I would not know that it was *the* cause of *this* headache. In the same way, I might find that Client 3 has frequent, intense, angry, and lengthy disputes with Client 3's spouse, and by a clever administration of applied behavior analysis, I might be able to reduce these disputes to near-zero levels, and find that Client 3's headaches now are much improved. I cite this third example, even knowing that two examples usually are enough for generalization, because I suspect that rather than generalizing, some of us are doing just the opposite with this third example: We are asserting that those inter-spouse disputes were indeed *the* cause of Client 3's headache. My problem is simply that Example 3 seems *formally* identical to Examples 1 and 2: In all three, a variable was manipulated to be different than it had been in the client's recent history, according to an ecological examination of that history; and in each example, that proved sufficient to yield experimental control over the headache under study, but not, for me, sufficient to establish that this variable was *the* cause of *this* headache rather than *a* possible cause of this headache and of headaches in general. Perhaps some of us like one variable better than another as *the* cause of *this* headache, but I cannot see how to be certain about that, not in retrospect.

Unless the operative stimulus control is that a cause ought to be something *ecologically natural?* Vitamin C, interestingly, is a natural component of many of the foods that we eat; by contrast, aspirin is a totaly artificial molecule. Is that why we are likely to be comfortable with the assertion that a lack of vitamin C is a cause of scurvy, while remaining uncomfortable with the parallel assertion that a lack of aspirin is a cause of headache? And is it a similar naturalness of interpersonal strife that makes it seem a reasonable candidate as a cause of headache, and an analogous unnaturalness of systematic relaxation as an instructed technique that makes us uncomfortable with the claim that its absence, like the absence of aspirin, is a cause of headache? Certainly, there is a valid distinction between events that occur naturally and events that occur only or mainly through our intervention; but is it a distinction worth great value in discriminating one kind of science from another? Is the discernment of causes already there so different a scientific venture from the discernment of cause in things that we make or provide, that it needs not only distinction but preference? I like to deal with causes, even if that is philosophically foolish, and I am willing to take refuge in the defensive terminology of functional relationships, if that avoids the philosophical objections, or simply to ignore the philosophical objections, if it doesn't.

Which returns me to the problem at hand: how to deal with *the* cause of *this* specific headache in a definitive way, rather than deal with only a possible cause of this particular headache and of headaches in general. The only headaches for which I ever have any certainty about *the* cause are the ones that I can cause myself through my own experimental manipulations; the ones already in existence seem to defy analysis for their *particular* cause.

If that's correct, then the analysis of *existing* organizations of behavior is inevitably an exercise in possible causes, not particular, specific, immediate causes; it is only the experimental *creation* of behavioral organizations that allows us a chance to know what specific immediate cause is at work in that process, and, by inference, could also be at work in similar situations, whether in the past, existing now, or in the future. The appropriate stimulus control is the distinction between analyzing already existing organizations of behavior by demonstrating what their causes *can* be, and analyzing what the specific causes of an organization of behavior *are* this time by experimentally creating it this time.

Applied behavior analysts deal mainly in trouble, and mainly with existing trouble; thus, when they analyze, they do indeed show merely what the causes of that kind of trouble *can* be, rather than definitively what they *are* this specific time. Most applied behavior analysts consider it unethical to experimentally create trouble, which, according to my argument, is the only way that they could be certain about the specific immediate cause of this particular troublesome organization of behavior. Thus, it is not the logic of their science, but the sociology of their science, that has them persistently dealing with *a* cause, one that can be applied to the present problem to affect a desirable behavior change, rather than with *the* cause that is responsible for the problem in, literally, the first place.

But pragmatically, the first place is no longer very important; it is the present place that counts now. When I argue here that a self-injurious child may not be behavior-disordered, but rather may be simply and naturally responsive to an environment that offers positive reinforcers that can be gained by that behavior, or negative reinforcers that can be avoided by that behavior, or no alternative ways of controlling the consequences that self-injurious behavior controls, I have no guarantee that any or all of these are causes in the first place. I know only that their manipulation now is likely to yield some amelioration of that self-injurious behavior, and that if it does, then our failure to so manipulate them is the cause of that self-injurious behavior continuing. That is a conservative concept of cause.

The underlying premise here is that in order to modify a behavior, you do not need to know its cause in the first place; and its obverse, which is that just because you can modify a behavior, that does not prove that you understand its cause in the first place. Recognition of this premise and its obverse is conservative, in that it encourages remediation in many cases where remediation is eminently attainable, rather than discouraging remediation for lack of an understanding of something called cause-in-the-first-place. It would be the opposite of conservative—it would be excruciatingly problematic—to assert that remediation is impossible in the absence of an understanding of cause in the first place. Imagine the efforts to prove an assertion like that! Imagine the intricacies of trying to explain away all the apparent exceptions to it in modern practice! Behavior-analytic logic conservatively does not require first causes, fortunately, and applied behavior analysis is sometimes effective, not in ordering disordered behavior, but in changing behavior that we complain about into behavior that we admire, or complaining behavior into admiring behavior. That is intimately connected to its conservatism; and that is the conservative thing to do while we wait to see if anyone else will ever clarify the first causes of these already existent problems, and ever prove that there is a concept of health, wholeness, or developmental integrity and propriety applicable to behavior problems, apart from the fact that behavior sometimes does not fit the arrangements that we wish it would.

Consider a straw example: The self-injurious behavior of some profoundly retarded, multiply handicapped institutionalized children has been postulated to result only epiphenomenally from the environmental contingencies that I have described; instead, it is assigned to fundamental processes within the self-injurious child, specifically, attributions of self-worthlessness. A bad enough self-image, perhaps, or a profound enough guilt, it has been argued, is causal to attempts at self-punishment and self-injury.

I cite this as a straw example, not because I constructed it to be self-destructive, but because I chose it as already manifestly self-destructive. Its implausibility makes it a good case for argument: Its content is absurd enough to be disbelieved, and thus not obscure the argument to follow, but its form as a potential case of environmental control of behavior is quite useful to a behavior-analytic approach. Free, then, from any tendency to believe this case, consider it simply as a possibility in cause and effect.

Could an internal, symbolic, and utterly private event cause external behavior such as self-injury? Surely, in principle; we all know that we sometimes plan our behavior at a totally internal, symbolic, and private level, and then act out those plans some time later. It is a manifestly possible and actual mechanism of cause-and-effect in behavior. In principle, profoundly retarded people could be engaging in self-injurious behavior as a moralistically logical outcome of an internal, symbolic, and private attribution of worthlessness to themselves. Those of us who teach them would be astounded at such capability in them, but that is a mere matter of factual plausibility. The form of cause-and-effect is sound, even if its content in this particular example is not.

But consider the reverse case: Could the systematic practice of self-injurious behavior be causal to an attribution of worthlessness? Surely; we often sum up a pattern of behavior in a few inductive symbols. If I spent much of my time trying to destroy myself, I might well notice that, and since I have a high rate of labeling response classes, I might label my own as worthlessness. Again, it is implausible that profoundly retarded people do that, but it is formally possible.

But also consider the orthogonal case: that attributions of worthlessness and systematic self-injury were both shaped by the same environmental source. Perhaps disgusted caretakers routinely teach some profoundly retarded people that they are worthless, and also routinely teach them that attention can be gained through self-injury more consistently than through any other avenue. Then they are both self-injurious and full of attributions of worthlessness, but neither has any causal relationship to the other—they are independent outcomes of common teaching agents who run at least these two curricula. But why would the caretakers systematically run both these curricula? Perhaps the profoundly retarded person's systematic self-injury is disgusting to the caretakers (who probably do not realize that they are its source), and out of that disgust the caretakers teach self-injurers that they are worthless.

I entertain these forms of cause and effect because, in my opinion, they are realistic forms often enough operative in behavior. Their content in this particular example was trivially easy to put aside, but the forms in which that content was made to operate are important cases, as forms. Conservative analysis might put these forms aside, not because their content in this case was absurd, but because their content in the typical case will be unobservable, and absent observation, we have no recourse other than to imagine or infer what their content might be in plausible cases. Some forms of conservatism are not satisfied with plausibility; they require provability. To the extent that internal processes operate in these forms of cause and effect, and to the extent that internal processes are unobservable, then these forms are useless to that kind of conservatism. Such conservatism marks the approach sometimes called methodological behaviorism (Skinner, 1974).

However, I mean to argue here (as elsewhere: Baer, 1982) that an even more profound level of conservatism will consider these forms of cause and effect, under certain quite specialized circumstances. In effect, I mean to argue from the stance of radical behaviorism—conservative radical behaviorism, of course (cf. Skinner, 1974). In that position, it is conservative to stipulate the existence of such private internal processes, because it is obvious that they exist and that they are behaviors. At least, it is obvious to me that they exist in me; the point then is not whether you believe me, but rather whether I am willing to suppose that what is real in me is very likely real in you, too. As an act of conservatism, I will so suppose. It would be drastic (not radical) to suppose differently. But the essence of conservatism will be to suppose further that these events, observable in me by me but not by you, are not different in kind from any other behavioral events that I possess and display for study by you. That is why I entertained all those cases of potential cause and effect: because the readily observable external behaviors that I and all of us possess certainly can enter into all those forms of cause and effect, and if they can, so can these unobservable ones.

The Law of Large Numbers implies that if they can, then, given sufficient opportunities, sometimes they will. Obviously, opportunity is more than sufficient; therefore, they do. Private, internal behaviors enter into all the cases and functions that we have shown that public behaviors can and do. However, note that the act of conservatism that confers on them all the powers and abilities of observable behaviors also limits them to only those powers. In a behavior-analytic view of the world, behaviors have no permanence or autonomy. The mechanisms that control them imply that they are always modifiable, if only those mechanisms can be got at. Thus, we may look for the cause of certain behaviors to be internal responses like attributions, self-instructions, and the like, but by the same token we must then look for the causes of those very internal responses themselves, and we must expect that their causes are similar in kind to the causes of more ordinary behaviors: Internal behaviors exist, they function in all possible positions within the forms of cause and effect, and they are just as subject to reinforcement, punishment, extinction, scheduling, stimulus control, and every other known mechanism of environmental control as are any other behaviors that we have ever studied. Thus, they can be just as effective as any other behaviors can be, and also just as ineffective. Just as we deny them autonomy from environmental control, so we deny them any other special attributes—other than difficult to observe. In particular, we suppose that inner events may mediate outer events, but no better, we assume, than any outer event could do, on the average.

Yet there remains the problem of unobservability. Only two things can be done with unobservable processes. One is to make inferences about them. Inference has never been a favored method in behavior-analytic logic, although it is not unknown. Skinner's (1957) book, *Verbal Behavior,* represents a totally inferential account of how language must function, if it is approached from a behavior-analytic standpoint. As one of my colleagues says of that analysis, "I can't imagine how it could be any other way." Neither can I, but I have no confidence that tomorrow someone may not imagine it quite a different way, and from the same standpoint.*

I, like many behavior analysts, prefer to deal with observables through observation; we are so distrustful of inference that we verge on refusing to consider private events beyond acknowledging their abstract existence, thereby almost sliding into methodological behaviorism. Fortunately, there is a supremely conservative second tactic in response to this problem: Rather than *infer* the nature of private events that might be mediating between external events, *teach* some mediating events that are likely to become private shortly after their acquisition. If we teach them, we know what their attributes are at the time; they may become unobservable later, and so we will not know, later, what they are like then—but we still shall know what we taught. The primal experiment here is to describe behavior as a set of interactions between observable stimuli and observable response, and then to teach in an observable way some currently observable potential mediators, and watch to see what difference that makes. Let them become unobservable, if they will; we still shall know what they were

---

* The analysis of language from a different standpoint has of course already been imagined in a very large variety of ways.

when we taught them, and what difference it made to do so, and that will constitute a quite fair analysis of behavior.

To teach is certainly one of the most conservative acts of behavior analysis that could be cited. True, to teach something that becomes unobservable, and so cannot be checked later to see if it is still what was taught or has become something different, is a trifle risqué—but the underlying tactic is conservative behavior analysis, and in logic offers an intriguing set of possibilities.

Applied behavior analysis has long used external change agents to alter undesirable behaviors of children. Inevitably, generalization of those changes has proven to be a problem. In the presence of the change agent, the behavior is different and desirable; in the absence of the change agent, it often is not. Those behaviors that the change agent changed directly are different and desirable; those that the change agent did not get to yet, often are not. Those stimulus controls that the change agent changed directly are different and desirable; those that the change agent did not get to yet often are not. A variety of methods are beginning to be explored for their power to do better than that (Stokes & Baer, 1977). One of them is the possibility of recruiting the child to do some of what the change agent does, but in the absence of the change agent, in any setting, and to every behavior, and at any time that is needful. In short, the tactic considered is to let the child mediate the generalization of the child's own behavior changes. All that that tactic requires is that the necessary mediating behaviors be taught to the child, and that *they* generalize as widely as needful.

Why should they? And why more than the behavior changes whose generalization they are supposed to mediate did? A not very behavior-analytic assumption is that if they are just the right kind of internal, typically private event, they might be especially good for that task. Conservatism suggests that they will be worth a try, a skeptical try, and that

- as long as the try centers on the teaching of those skills rather than the inference of their character and function, and
- as long as the teaching is done with the best teaching technology that applied behavior analysis knows, and
- as long as competent experimental designs are used to see what difference it makes to do so, and
- as long as any differences that it makes are conceptualized and measured directly as behaviors and behavior changes,

then it will be applied behavior analysis even if it does go invisible at one crucial point. And if the results are exciting, then it will be exciting applied behavior analysis as well. Meichenbaum and his colleagues have been doing this kind of research for some years (Meichenbaum, 1977; Meichenbaum & Goodman, 1971).

I offer in conclusion the notion that applied behavior analysis is a conservative approach to childhood behavior disorders. It is conservative in that it does not consider them disorders; conservative in that it includes in their analysis the analysis of the behavior of others who do think of them as disorders; conservative in that its orientation is toward the workable current-environmental mechanisms that may contribute to their change (when analysis indicates change); conservative in its standards of proof; and conservative in its admiration for functional teaching as an essence of analysis. I offer these characteristics of behavior-analytic thought in the same conservative spirit that traditional researchers offer the null hypothesis: If you want to go beyond this characterization of the process, you will have to show something that this characterization cannot understand and control, and that some alternative can both understand and control. In the spirit of single-subject design, Type 1 errors should be made improbable. Meanwhile, we shall continue to expand the capabilities of our null hypothesis—conservatively, of course.

REFERENCES

BAER, D. M. (1982). Applied behavior analysis. In G. T. Wilson & C. M. Franks (Eds.), *Contemporary behavior therapy*. New York: Guilford Press.

DEITZ, S. M., & BAER, D. M. (1982, May). *Is technology a dirty word?* Paper presented at the meeting of the Association for Behavior Analysis, Milwaukee.

MEICHENBAUM, D. H. (1977). *Cognitive-behavior modification*. New York: Plenum.

MEICHENBAUM, D. H., & GOODMAN, J. (1971). Training impulsive children to talk to themselves: A means of developing self-control. *Journal of American Psychology*, 77(2), 115-126.

SKINNER, B. F. (1957). *Verbal behavior*. New York: Appleton-Century-Crofts.

SKINNER, B. F. (1974). *About behaviorism*. New York: Knopf.

STOKES, T. F., & BAER, D. M. (1977). An implicit technology of generalization. *Journal of Applied Behavior Analysis, 10*, 349-367.

3

A Cognitive-Behavioral Perspective of Child Psychopathology: Implications for Assessment and Training

DONALD H. MEICHENBAUM,
LINDA A. BREAM, and JANICE S. COHEN

In recent years, both psychology and behavior therapy have been influenced by the emergence, or should we say the reemergence, of the important roles of cognitive and affective processes in understanding and treating behavior disorders. A byproduct of what Dember (1974) has called a "cognitive revolution" in psychology has been the development of a cognitive-behavioral perspective of behavior disorders and treatment. In this chapter we will illustrate this cognitive-behavioral perspective as it applies to childhood disorders and, more specifically, the instance of the socially withdrawn child.

Although some beginning steps in this research approach have been undertaken, a great deal more understanding is required before effective interventions can be developed. Before we consider childhood disorders, let us briefly look at the basic tenets or working framework of a cognitive-behavioral perspective and its implications for assessment and treatment.

COGNITIVE-BEHAVIORAL PERSPECTIVE

1) A cognitive-behavioral perspective embraces a transactional model of stress and coping as proposed by Richard Lazarus (Lazarus, 1981; Lazarus & Launier, 1978) and John Mason (1971). According to the transactional model, stress resides neither in the situation nor in the person. Instead, stress depends on the transaction of the individual in the situation. The individual's perception of both the stressfulness of the event and his or her ability to cope with events ultimately defines stress.

2) A cognitive-behavioral perspective emphasizes the interdependence of several concurrent processes in understanding behavior. These processes include thoughts, feelings, behaviors, and the perception of their intra- and interpersonal consequences. This interdependence has been highlighted in Bandura's (1978) "reciprocal determinism" model, which underscores the concurrent influences on behavior of several intra- and interpersonal processes. Accordingly, the cognitive-behavioral perspective argues that it is not the consequences of behavior per se that automatically influence behavior, but rather how the individual appraises such consequences.

3) One concurrent process which has been highlighted in the cognitive-behavioral perspective is the individual's thoughts. In referring to the role of the individual's thoughts, the cognitive-behavior theorist distinguishes between cognitive events, cognitive processes, and cognitive structures. Since these distinctions have relevance for an understanding of childhood disorders, a brief description of each will help. (See Meichenbaum & Gilmore, in press, and Turk & Speers, 1983, for a fuller discussion of the role of cognition.)

Cognitive events refer to conscious thoughts and images that occur in an individual's stream of consciousness or can be readily retrieved upon request. Beck (1976) has referred to them as "automatic thoughts" and Meichenbaum (1977) has described them as "internal dialogue." Cognitive events incorporate, among other things, attributions, expectancies, evaluations of self or task, and task-irrelevant thoughts. Such automatic cognitive events are not limited to cognitions, but may involve images, symbolic "words," gestures, and *their accompanying affect*. These cognitive events may at times be affectively laden or constitute what Zajonc (1980) has described as "hot" as compared to "cold" cognitions.

Cognitive events (or what Langer, 1978, has called "mindful" behavior) are likely to occur: 1) during the construction and integration of new thought and action structures, e.g., learning a new motor skill; 2) when an individual has to exercise choices and judgments as in uncertain or novel situations, e.g., covert trial and error conditions or when one's plans are interrupted; and 3) when an individual anticipates and/or experiences an intense emotional experience.

Cognitive processes are those processes that shape, transform, and construct mental representations into schemes of experience and action. They include search and storage mechanisms, inferential processes, and retrieval processes. Subsumed under this topic are such processes as metacognitions (Flavell, 1979), mental heuristics (Kahneman & Tversky, 1973), confirmatory biases (Frank, 1974; Snyder, 1981), maladaptive cognitions (e.g., distorted interpretations, unwarranted catastrophic anticipations, self-denigrating ideation), and disruptive feelings (e.g., anxiety, depression, hopelessness). These cognitive and affective processes may operate in an automatic scripted fashion (Abelson, 1976), influencing which events are attended to, how events are appraised, and which events are stored and retrieved.

Cognitive structures refer to tacit assumptions and beliefs that give rise to habitual ways of construing the self and the world. The individual's personal schemata, current concerns, hidden agendas, and personal goals influence the way information is processed and the way behavior is organized. George Kelly (1969) anticipated the current interest in cognitive structures in his personal construct theory. As Kelly noted, cognitive structures act as perceptual sets which serve a "gating function." It is important to appreciate that each cognitive structure or schema embodies both an ideational component and an affective component. Not only is information coded and stored, but so is affect (Bower, 1981). Such schemata operate like Kuhn's (1970) paradigms and Polanyi's (1958) tacit knowledge in influencing behavior.

Now that we have briefly introduced some of the major propositions and concepts of a cognitive-behavioral perspective we can illustrate their operation in explaining psychopathology. The first example we have chosen comes from adult psychopathology, since most research has been done on this population. Although the example involves adult abnormal behavior, we believe that the same principles can have heuristic value in understanding childhood psychopathology. Thus, we will first consider the adult disorder of unipolar depression and then focus on the childhood disorder of social withdrawal. These two examples were chosen because we feel the research findings lend themselves to a cognitive-behavioral analysis. We do *not* mean to suggest that there is a developmental link between these two disorders.

UNIPOLAR DEPRESSION

One of the most researched problems in adult psychopathology is that of depression. The picture that is beginning to emerge is as follows:

1) An adult who is depressed is characterized by a dysphoric mood, sadness, feelings of helplessness and hopelessness, and a sense of victimization (i.e., a sense of not being able to control one's feelings and thoughts).

2) Research by Teasdale (1983) and Bower (1981) indicates that a depressed mood affects one's cognitive processes in terms of slowing down the speed of information processing, selectively recalling negative events, and fostering a negative attributional style (i.e., more characterological self-blame).

3) Another characteristic of a depressed individual is that he or she has a depressing impact on others. The work of Coyne (1982) and Gotlib (1982) indicates that depressed individuals tend to turn others off, leading to social avoidance and rejection, which confirms the depressed individual's initial beliefs of worthlessness. In fact, in many instances, depressed individuals have social skills deficits (Rehm, 1977) and they often tend to perceive the consequences of their actions more harshly than do non-depressed individuals (Lewinsohn, Mischel, Chaplin, & Barton, 1980).

4) These social consequences confirm the individual's "depressogenic" assumptions and cognitive schemata of abandonment, loss, and failure. These current concerns contribute to a thinking style that may further distort events in order to confirm their previous depressive bias. Thus, a self-confirmatory bias develops, whereby depressed individuals search the past, present, and future to confirm their depressive state (Beck, 1976). Moreover, depressed individuals often help to create the very environment that confirms their depressed condition.

In summary, adult depression illustrates that cognitive structures, processes, events, affective states, behavioral acts, and their perceived consequences interact to maintain a vicious, self-defeating cycle. Depressed feelings and thoughts have an impact on the client's behavior, which often leads to inactivity that can, in turn, contribute to biochemical changes and further exacerbate the depression (Akiskal &

McKinney, 1975). According to this model, it would be difficult to argue that any set of factors—biochemical processes, thoughts, feelings, behavior and their consequences—are *the* cause of depression. Instead, one should attempt to assess the contribution of each component process to the disordered behavior.

Following from this analysis, a cognitive-behavioral treatment approach is designed to: (a) make the client aware of this automatic interdependent maladaptive process; (b) teach the client to interrupt this sequence; (c) help the client to produce incompatible thoughts, feelings, and behaviors; and (d) perform "personal experiments" which lead to data which is incompatible with one's prior expectations and provides "evidence" contradictory to one's cognitive structures. Change in one's cognitive structures is most likely to occur by discovering through enactive experiences that old cognitive structures are unwarranted; and the adoption of new, more adaptive structures is rewarding. Some clients may need skills training and support in conducting such enactive experiences or personal experiments. The cognitive-behavioral treatment approach has been described by Beck, Rush, Shaw, and Emery (1979), Meichenbaum (1977) and Turk, Meichenbaum, and Genest (1983).

Although a great deal more research is needed to explicate the nature of adult depression, this example provides a useful framework for understanding childhood disorders. How do cognitive-affective structures, processes, events, feelings, behaviors and environmental events interact in the case of childhood disorders? We will try to answer this question for the socially withdrawn child.

THE SOCIALLY WITHDRAWN CHILD

The study of childhood psychopathology has increasingly focused upon the role of children's peer relationships. There is evidence to indicate that early peer difficulties are predictive of later social and psychological maladjustment (e.g., Cowen, Pederson, Babigan, Izzo, & Trost, 1973; Roff, Sells, & Golden, 1972) and that one's peer status is quite stable over time (Coie & Dodge, 1983). As Putallaz and Gottman (1983) indicate, children who are unpopular (neglected and/or rejected by their peers) are more likely to be low achievers in school, experience more learning difficulties, to drop out of school, and to experience a number of subsequent problems (e.g., higher rates of juvenile delinquency in adolescence, and higher rates of mental health problems in adulthood). In citing these studies, Putallaz and Gottman warn that, since these outcome studies are often subject to methodological problems, one must be cautious in interpreting correlational data (low social status in childhood and subsequent negative outcomes) as being causative. Even though Putallaz and Gottman express such cautions, they indicate that 10% to 15% of children during grade school are *not* liked by peers and face the possibility of continued neglect and/or rejection. In a similar vein, Asher, Hymel, and Renshaw (1983) surveyed over 500 third-through sixth-grade children using a self-report measure of loneliness. Ten percent of these children reported feelings of loneliness and social dissatisfaction.

Such survey data take on clinical significance when one considers the importance assigned to peer relationships and friendships in the development of social adjustment. A number of developmental theorists (e.g., Piaget, Sullivan, Hartup) have viewed friendships as the arena in which a child learns a number of important concepts (e.g., reciprocity, cooperation) and interpersonal skills (e.g., perspective-taking, social problem-solving, conflict resolution).

As the data on peer relationships accumulate, there is a growing appreciation of the variety of types of social problems children may exhibit. More specifically, when sociometric procedures are used to target children, it is important to highlight the distinction between the child who is ignored or neglected by peers and the child who is rejected or actively disliked (Asher & Hymel, 1981). Recent research indicates that these two (sociometrically defined) groups of children manifest different behavioral styles with different social consequences (Coie, Dodge, & Coppotelli, 1982; Coie & Kupersmidt, in press; Dodge, in press). Until recently, both the neglected and rejected child have been subsumed under the general label of the unpopular child. Furthermore, researchers have also distinguished between socially-at-risk children who have been targeted behaviorally (e.g., socially withdrawn children with low levels of peer interaction) and those who have been identified by means of sociometric measures (Rubin, 1982). We will focus on the child who experiences problems both of social withdrawal and of social neglect.

Consider the case of 11-year-old Ellen M. who was brought to the clinic by her mother because of her concern that Ellen did not have friends, and was extremely shy and isolated. Ellen tended to avoid others, remained on the periphery of social activities, and felt lonely. Her efforts to make friends were often ignored by her peers. In school, Ellen did not have any particular academic problems, but her teacher expressed concern about Ellen's inability to establish and maintain friendships. Both sociometric and interview data reflected a child who was socially neglected. (See Bierman, 1983a, for an example of such an interview.)

The next step in the cognitive-behavioral analysis was an assessment of the adequacy of Ellen's behavioral repertoire of social skills; i.e., her ability to initiate interactions, to maintain ongoing interactions, and to resolve conflicts. A number of observational studies in both natur-alistic and analogue situations have indicated that unpopular children: (a) interact less frequently with peers; (b) make fewer initiations to, and requests of, peers; and (c) disagree more, call attention to them-selves, state opinions, and behave more negatively (Hops, 1983).

Illustrative of these findings are the sequential behavior analyses of unpopular and popular children's interactions as they attempt to enter dyads of popular and unpopular children. Putallaz and Gottman (1981) found that when popular children disagree they would typically cite a general rule as the basis for disagreements, and then provide an acceptable alternative action for the other child. In contrast, unpopular children would follow peer disagreements by stating a prohibition very specific to previous acts of the other child, without providing an alter-native action for that child. Interestingly, these findings were qualified by the status of the peer groups which the child entered. The same initiating behavior was responded to differently by different groups (i.e., popular or unpopular dyads). Thus, in order to be successful in gaining entry into a group, a child must learn to consider the frame of reference of the group. Moreover, Putallaz (in press) reported that the ability to accurately perceive and contribute to the group's ongoing activities correlates with subsequent social status. The findings of Pu-tallaz and Gottman indicate the complexity and sensitivity involved in social skills.

A cognitive-behavioral perspective, however, goes beyond the focus upon overt social skills and peer status by asking what factors underlie the child's inability to manifest the desirable social behavior. Does the child have a deficit in social knowledge and/or do affective, cognitive, and interpersonal factors interfere with the child emitting social skills that are indeed in his or her repertoire?

Several investigators (Gottman, Gonso, & Rasmussen, 1975; Ladd & Oden, 1979) have reported that children who were sociometrically identified as being unpopular tended to have non-normative ideas about friendship, reciprocity, and about helping friends. Asher and Renshaw (1981) found that popular children's ideas were more affective and relationship-enhancing than those of unpopular children. Recent work by Renshaw and Asher (in press) indicates that unpopular children have different goals for social interaction. Specifically, they found that in a situation involving the maintenance of a friendship, low status children were less positive-outgoing in their goal orientation and suggested avoidance strategies almost exclusively. These processes were also evident in the case of Ellen.

A clinical interview, a role-playing assessment, and an assessment of social problem-solving skills (Elias, Larcen, Zlotlow, & Chinsky, 1978; Schwartz & Gottman, 1976) indicated that Ellen had a basic knowledge of how to establish friendships, but she failed to generate such strategies whenever social rejection was likely. In fact, Ellen reported that she would spend much of her time in class watching the most popular girls. She would then practice these social behaviors at home in front of the mirror. Ellen indicated, however, that if she attempted to implement such behaviors with her classmates, as her mother suggested, it would not be "natural." As she noted: "I would be fooling others. Deep down I am not like that." She felt that if she did try she would only be doing it for her mother or for her teacher. Moreover, on the one occasion when Ellen tried the practiced social skills and she met with some acceptance, she felt that the "other girls were only trying to be nice to me" and "they must have felt sorry for me and they didn't really mean being nice." These comments reflect Ellen's self-defeating avoidant-engendering pattern of attributions in social situations. She had the tendency to appraise events in terms of her prior expectations and current concerns revolving around a fear of social rejection. This preoccupation contributed to an avoidance and vigilance about social situations in which possible rejection may take place.

Ellen's case is consistent with a burgeoning literature which suggests that, in order to understand the nature of the deficits of socially withdrawn children, one should go beyond the nature of their overt behavioral repertoire and consider the role of cognitive and affective processes. For example, Ames, Ames, and Garrison (1977) found that low status children attributed social success to external causes and social failure to internal, personal causes, while the reverse was true for high status children. More recently, Goetz and Dweck (1980) found that children who attributed social rejection to internal, stable characteristics ("It's hard for me to make friends," "I can't do anything right") were less likely to persist after an initial rejection. Similarly, Dodge, Glassey, and Buchsbaum (1983) reported that neglected children misattributed hostility to accidental and prosocial acts of others and were more likely to respond to peer provocations with withdrawal. The potential significance of attributional processes contributing to social withdrawal was further suggested by Wheeler and Ladd (1982) who developed a children's social self-efficacy scale. In their preliminary results they found that the degree of self-efficacy is negatively related to anxiety and moderately, but positively, related to peer ratings of social influence and positive play nominations.

In *summary,* the research on children with social problems suggests that such processes as cognitive-affective structures, processes, events, behavioral acts and the interpretation of social consequences all contribute to inadequate social performance. (See Ladd & Mize, in press, for a discussion of other supportive studies that implicate the role of cognitive and affective processes contributing to social withdrawal in children.) The cognitive-behavioral transactional model that was offered to explain adult depression may indeed be useful in understanding socially withdrawn children. For example, in the case of Ellen her conflicting personal goals of wanting to make friends combined with her overriding fear of social rejection colored how she appraised situations and influenced her approach and avoidance behavior. These cognitive structures influenced her cognitive processing (i.e., attributional style, selective appraisal of past, present, and future events) of social situations. Such feelings and thoughts interfered with her social repertoire and these thoughts, in turn, came to act as self-fulfilling prophecies, leading to the very rejection that she feared. She had a confirmatory bias for social rejection and appraised events accordingly. She had a penchant to interpret the consequences of social interactions in a negative manner and to explain away positive social interactions. Such perceptions contributed to the avoidance of social interactions that would provide the very opportunities needed to change her behavior. Moreover, Ellen's social reputation in the peer group further reduced the likelihood of successful social experiences that could undo this negative cycle.

IMPLICATION FOR TREATMENT

The previous section indicated that the first step in formulating a treatment plan for the socially withdrawn child is the need to carefully determine the contributions of several concurrent processes to the performance deficit. Such an analysis provides critical information needed to tailor the intervention to the needs of each child. For example, Furman (1980) and Bierman (1982) have noted that the nature and effectiveness of social skills training are influenced by developmental changes in (a) the children's knowledge and conceptualization of social events, (b) the importance of peer interactions, and (c) the structure and importance of the peer group. Additionally, in individualizing an intervention program, the trainer must take sex differences into consideration. For example, Waldrop and Halverson (1975) reported that girls tend to form more intense relationships involving close friendships and low energy play, as compared to boys who tend to be at the opposite end of these dimensions. Findings such as these highlight the need for the cognitive-behavior therapist to take into consideration developmental, sex, and sociocultural differences.

In addition to analyzing the nature of the child's overt behaviors that need to be trained, as has been suggested earlier, the cognitive-behavior therapist should be sensitive to the role of cognitive factors (e.g., social knowledge, attributional style, appraisal process, social problem-solving skills) and affective factors (e.g., sense of helplessness, depression, anxiety) that may contribute to and exacerbate inadequate performance. One may obtain the same behavioral deficit of social withdrawal for a variety of reasons, and social skills training programs may prove effective for many different reasons. Social skills training with children (i.e., teaching them entry behaviors, cooperation, asking positive questions, and so forth) may help "unpopular" children (a) acquire new goals for social interaction, (b) gain confidence in their ability, and (c) learn to monitor their own and others' social behaviors (Asher & Renshaw, 1981; Dweck, 1981; Renshaw & Asher, in press). Thus, interdependent processes may contribute to performance deficits, and interventions in any one area (e.g., skills training) may have an impact or mediate change by affecting other concurrent processes.

A second major consideration in formulating a training program is to appreciate the limitations of previous efforts at intervention, especially the difficulty in obtaining generalization of treatment effects across setting and tasks, and over time. Several investigators (Brown & Campione, 1978; Meichenbaum, 1983; Stokes & Baer, 1977) have cautioned trainers that they should not lament the fact that they do not obtain generalization, but instead they should build generalization into the training regimen. Interestingly, even though these authors are coming from different theoretical perspectives and research areas (metacognitive development, cognitive-behavior modification, and operant conditioning, respectively), they suggest similar guidelines for achieving generalization. Although space does not permit a detailed consideration of these factors, some appreciation of them indicates their importance in any intervention program.

Table 1 summarizes the various factors that should be considered in any training program in order to increase the likelihood of generalized improvement. These guidelines underscore the need to ensure that the referred child collaborates in the treatment intervention. The focus of various coaching programs has been on teaching specific social skills, with little attention being paid to "implementation" factors. There is a need to ensure that the referred child:

1) understands the reasons why he or she is being seen and perceives that he or she has a problem;
2) collaborates in the selection of the skills to be worked on;
3) appreciates how the skills that will be worked on in the clinic will be helpful in changing behaviors in the criterion situations;

TABLE 1

Guidelines to Consider in Developing a Training Program

---

1) *Analyze target behaviors.* Conduct both a performance and situation analysis. Identify component processes and capacity requirements to perform target behaviors.
2) *Assessment.* Assess for client's existing strategies, behavioral competencies, and affect-laden thoughts, images, and feelings that may inhibit performance.
3) *Collaborate.* Have client collaborate in the analysis of the problem and in the development, implementation, and evaluation of the training package.
4) *Select training tasks carefully.* Make training tasks similar to the criterion.
5) *Training.* Ensure that the component skills needed to perform in the criterion situation are in the client's repertoire and then teach metacognitive or executive planning skills.
6) *Feedback.* Ensure that the client receives and recognizes feedback about the usefulness of the training procedures.
7) *Generalize.* Make the need and means for generalizing explicit. Don't expect generalization—train for it.
8) *Multiple trials.* When possible, train in multiple settings with multiple tasks and trainers. Have clients engage in multiple graded assignments in clinic and in vivo.
9) *Relapse prevention.* Anticipate and incorporate possible and real failures into the training program.
10) *Termination.* Make the termination of training performance-based, not time-based. Include follow-through booster sessions and follow-up assessments.

---

4) considers when and how he or she will practice these cognitive, affective, interpersonal skills in other situations (i.e., metacognitive training in the form of self-monitoring, self-interrogation, self-evaluation, etc.);

5) anticipates and reacts constructively to possible negative consequences (relapse-prevention training).

In short, the cognitive-behavioral treatment approach recognizes from the outset the complex nature of the social skills that are to be taught and the transactional nature of the intervention. Treatment should go beyond performance-enhancement procedures and focus on cognitive and affective processes. Moreover, consistent with the transactional nature of a cognitive-behavioral approach, intervention should extend beyond the socially withdrawn child to include, whenever possible, the relevant peer group.

Efforts at treating socially withdrawn children have included coaching, behavioral rehearsal, structured opportunities to practice, and feedback (e.g., Berler, Gross, & Drabman, 1982; Van Hasselt, Hersen, Whitehill, & Bellack, 1979). Such behaviorally based interventions have not focused on the role of cognitive and affective processes. This oversight may have contributed to the limited efficacy of social skills training programs (Asher & Renshaw, 1981). When social skills training programs result in changes in the behavior of the socially withdrawn child, often these gains do *not* extend to changes in the perceived social status of the withdrawn child (e.g., LaGreca & Santogrossi, 1980). As Bierman (1981) and Putallaz (1982) indicate, the peer group often responds to the socially withdrawn child's former reputation rather than to his or her present level of social skills. The work of Dodge (Dodge, 1980; in press) further supports the importance of considering a child's acquired social reputation and indicates that these reputations emerge over time and become increasingly stable with age.

These reputation studies highlight the need to develop interventions that focus on the child's peer group as well as on the individual child. Although the evidence for the effectiveness of involving the peer group in treatment of children with social problems is *not* very strong (Putallaz, 1982), recent efforts by Bierman (1981, 1983b) are encouraging. Following in the tradition of the Sherifs (1964), who noted the potential benefits of establishing superordinate goals, Bierman was able to involve peers in tasks with unpopular children (e.g., creating skits, making videotapes, and so forth). The combined effects of skills coaching and peer involvement improved the social acceptance of the unpopular children. Indeed, skills coaching studies that have included the re-hearsal of trained skills with a peer have been the most effective in changing peer sociometric status (Oden & Asher, 1977; Ladd, 1981).

Another related approach to training has been to structure the un-popular child's social environment to maximize the opportunities for social interactions (see Furman, Rahe, & Hartup, 1979). These at-tempts have included pairing the unpopular child with a younger peer or introducing the unpopular child to a new, unfamiliar peer group where he or she has no preestablished reputation. Such opportunities provide the unpopular child with an occasion to perform "personal experiments" in order to try out social skills that he or she has been working on. The potential benefits of such interventions are indicated by Coie and Kupersmidt's (in press) findings that neglected children who were perceived as shy in familiar groups achieved a more favorable status in unfamiliar groups. More work needs to be done to integrate and combine the different approaches to training. Moreover, the rel-evance of particular treatment approaches at different developmental levels needs to be clarified.

In addition to teaching Ellen the relevant skills and providing her with opportunities to practice newly acquired skills, the cognitive be-haviorist would include efforts at helping her (a) develop a more mature conception of friendship (give and take reciprocal relationships, per-spective-taking), and (b) learn to anticipate and handle relapse (i.e., an appreciation that negative consequences and rejection are natural dimensions of social interactions). Much emphasis should be placed on helping her assess personal goals and the need to establish synchrony with the group; that is, learning to act in a manner that is consistent with the ongoing group activity. The need to determine the group's frame of reference has been noted by Putallaz (1982). In short, training is designed to make the unpopular child aware of the sequence of processes that trigger, maintain, and exacerbate withdrawal and to learn incompatible responses. From a cognitive-behavioral perspective, the inclusion of performance-based efforts provides the data whereby the child and trainer can work together to evaluate the significance of such social consequences for the child's cognitive-affective struc-tures, processes, and events.

Thus, the circle is complete. The transactional model (involving multiple concurrent processes) that was offered to understand the na-ture of behavior disorders such as social withdrawal provides the framework for understanding behavior change. The challenge for investigators with a cognitive-behavioral perspective is to develop sensitive and reliable assessment instruments to tap each of the processes described in this chapter and to demonstrate how they interact and change. How do successful (rewarding) performance-based efforts contribute to changes in self-efficacy, attributions, and expectations? How many and what type of successful interpersonal interactions are needed to change personal goals and cognitive structures? How does one account for the success of social skills training when it does indeed occur? Until sensitive "dipstick" measures of multiple processes have been developed and the interdependence of the processes demonstrated, the present cognitive-behavioral model offers only a promising agenda for future research.

The transactional model and the cognitive-behavioral perspective (e.g., à la case of unipolar depression) provide a heuristic framework for understanding childhood disorders. In fact, we could have attempted a similar analysis of other childhood disorders. For example, the work on hyperactive-aggressive children and learning-disabled children has similarly implicated the role of personal goals, social knowledge, metacognitive deficits, attributional style, appraisal processes, interpersonal style, perception of social consequences, peer interactions, and parental factors (e.g., marital discord, insularity, maternal depression) as contributing to, maintaining, and exacerbating maladaptive child behaviors. The challenge is to integrate these various processes into a theoretically testable model.

References

ABELSON, R. P. (1976). Script processing in attitude formation and decision making. In J. Carroll & J. Payne (Eds.), *Cognition and social behavior*. Hillsdale, NJ: Erlbaum.

AKISKAL, H., & McKINNEY, W. (1975). Overview of recent research in depression. *Archives of General Psychiatry, 32*, 285-305.

AMES, R., AMES, C., & GARRISON, W. (1977). Children's causal ascriptions for positive and negative interpersonal outcomes. *Psychological Reports, 41*, 595-602.

ASHER, S. R., & HYMEL, S. (1981). Children's social competence in peer relations: Sociometric and behavioral assessment. In J. D. Wine & M. D. Syme (Eds.), *Social competence*. New York: Guilford Press.

ASHER, S. R., HYMEL, S., & RENSHAW, P. (1983). *Loneliness in children*. Unpublished manuscript, University of Illinois, Champaign.

ASHER, S., & RENSHAW, P. (1981). Children without friends: Social knowledge and social skills training. In S. Asher & J. Gottman (Eds.), *The development of children's friendships*. New York: Cambridge University Press.

BANDURA, A. (1978). The self-system in reciprocal determinism. *American Psychologist, 33*, 344-358.

BECK, A. (1976). *Cognitive therapy and the emotional disorders.* New York: International Universities Press.

BECK, A., RUSH, A., SHAW, B., & EMERY, G. (1979). *Cognitive therapy of depression.* New York: Guilford Press.

BERLER, E., GROSS, A., & DRABMAN, R. (1982). Social skills training with children: Proceed with caution. *Journal of Applied Behavior Analysis, 15,* 41-53.

BIERMAN, K. (1981). *Enhancing generalization of social skills training with peer involvement and superordinate goals.* Paper presented at the meeting of the Society for Research in Child Development, Boston.

BIERMAN, K. (1982). *Social skills training from a developmental perspective.* Paper presented at the meeting of the Association for the Advancement of Behavior Therapy, Los Angeles.

BIERMAN, K. (1983a, April). *A standardized child interview to assess social competence and peer relationships.* Paper presented at the meeting of the Society for Research in Child Development, Detroit.

BIERMAN, K. (1983b, April). *The effects of social skills training on the interactions of unpopular and popular peers engaged in cooperative tasks.* Paper presented at the meeting of the Society for Research in Child Development, Detroit.

BOWER, G. (1981). Mood and memory. *American Psychologist, 36,* 129-148.

BROWN, A., & CAMPIONE, J. (1978). Permissible inference from the outcome of training studies in cognitive development research. *Quarterly Newsletter of the Institute for Comparative Human Development, 2,* 46-53.

COIE, J., & DODGE, K. (1983). Continuities and change in children's social status: A five year longitudinal study. *Merrill-Palmer Quarterly, 29,* 261-282.

COIE, J., DODGE, K., & COPPOTELLI, H. (1982). Dimensions and types of social status: A cross-age perspective. *Developmental Psychology, 18,* 557-570.

COIE, J., & KUPERSMIDT, J. (in press). A behavioral analysis of emerging social status in boys' groups. *Child Development.*

COWEN, E. L., PEDERSON, A., BABIGAN, H., IZZO, L. D., & TROST, M. A. (1973). Long-term follow-up of early detected vulnerable children. *Journal of Consulting and Clinical Psychology, 41,* 438-446.

COYNE, J. (1982). A critique of cognitions as causal entities with particular reference to depression. *Cognitive Therapy and Research, 6,* 3-13.

DEMBER, W. (1974). Motivation and the cognitive revolution. *American Psychologist, 29,* 161-168.

DODGE, K. (1980). Social cognition and children's aggressive behavior. *Child Development, 51,* 162-170.

DODGE, K. (in press). Behavioral antecedents of peer social status. *Child Development.*

DODGE, K., GLASSEY, R. M., & BUCHSBAUM, K. (1983). *The assessment of intention-cue detection skills in children: Implications for developmental psychopathology.* Unpublished manuscript, Indiana University.

DWECK, C. (1981). Social cognitive processes in children's friendships. In S. Asher & J. Gottman (Eds.), *The development of children's friendships.* New York: Cambridge University Press.

ELIAS, M., LARCEN, S., ZLOTLOW, S., & CHINSKY, J. (1978). *An innovative measure of children's cognitions in problematic interpersonal situations.* Paper presented at the meeting of the American Psychological Association, Toronto.

FLAVELL, J. (1979). Metacognition and cognitive monitoring: A new area of cognitive-developmental inquiry. *American Psychologist, 34,* 906-911.

FRANK, J. (1974). *Persuasion and healing* (2nd ed.). New York: Schocken Books.

FURMAN, W. (1980). Promoting social development: Developmental implications for treatment. In B. Lahey & A. Kazdin (Eds.), *Advances in clinical child psychology* (Vol. 3). New York: Plenum Press.

FURMAN, W., RAHE, D., & HARTUP, W. W. (1979). Rehabilitation of socially-withdrawn preschool children through mixed-age and same-age socialization. *Child Development, 50,* 915-922.

GOETZ, T., & DWECK, C. (1980). Learned helplessness in social situations. *Journal of Personality and Social Psychology, 39,* 246-255.

GOTLIB, I. (1982). Self-reinforcement and depression in interpersonal interaction: The role of performance level. *Journal of Abnormal Psychology, 91,* 3-13.

GOTTMAN, J., GONSO, J., & RASMUSSEN, B. (1975). Social interaction, social competence and friendship in children. *Child Development, 46,* 709-718.

HOPS, H. (1983). Children's social competence and skill: Current research practices and future directions. *Behavior Therapy, 14,* 3-18.

KAHNEMAN, D., & TVERSKY, A. (1973). On the psychology of prediction. *Psychological Review, 80,* 237-251.

KELLY, G. (1969). Personal construct theory and the psychotherapeutic interview. In B. Maher (Ed.), *Clinical psychology and personality: The selected papers of George Kelly.* New York: Wiley.

KUHN, T. (1970). *The structure of scientific revolutions.* Chicago: University of Chicago Press.

LADD, G. W. (1981). Effectiveness of a social learning method for enhancing children's social interaction and peer acceptance. *Child Development, 52,* 171-178.

LADD, G., & MIZE, J. (in press). A cognitive-social learning model of social skills training. *Psychological Review.*

LADD, G., & ODEN, S. (1979). The relationship between peer acceptance and children's ideas about helpfulness. *Child Development, 50,* 402-408.

LaGRECA, A. M., & SANTOGROSSI, D. A. (1980). Social skills training with elementary school children: A behavioral group approach. *Journal of Consulting and Clinical Psychology, 48,* 220-227.

LANGER, E. (1978). Rethinking the role of thought in social interaction. In J. Harvey, W. Ickes, & R. Kidd (eds.), *New directions in attribution research* (Vol. 2). Hillsdale, NJ: Erlbaum.

LAZARUS, R. (1981). The stress and coping paradigm. In C. Eisdorfer (Ed.), *Models for clinical psychopathology.* New York: Spectrum Press.

LAZARUS, R., & LAUNIER, R. (1978). Stress-related transactions between persons and environment. In L. Pervin & M. Lewis (Eds.), *Perspectives in interactional psychology.* New York: Plenum Press.

LEWINSOHN, P., MISCHEL, W., CHAPLIN, W., & BARTON, R. (1980). Social competence and depression: The role of illusory self-perceptions? *Journal of Abnormal Psychology, 89,* 203-212.

MASON, J. A. (1971). Reevaluation of the concept "non-specificity" in stress theory. *Journal of Psychiatric Research, 8,* 323-333.

MEICHENBAUM, D. (1977). *Cognitive behavior modification: An integrative approach.* New York: Plenum Press.

MEICHENBAUM, D. (1983). Teaching thinking: A cognitive-behavioral perspective. In J. Segal, S. Chipman & R. Glaser (Eds.), *Thinking and learning skills* (Vol. 2). Hillsdale, NJ: Erlbaum.

MEICHENBAUM, D., & GILMORE, B. (in press). Resistance: From a cognitive-behavioral perspective. In P. Wachtel (Ed.), *Resistance in psychodynamic and behavioral therapies.* New York: Plenum Press.

ODEN, S., & ASHER, S. (1977). Coaching children in social skills for friendship making. *Child Development, 48,* 495-506.

POLANYI, M. (1958). *Personal knowledge: Towards a post-critical philosophy.* Chicago: University of Chicago Press.

PUTALLAZ, M. (1982). *The importance of the peer group for successful intervention.* Paper presented at the meeting of the Association for the Advancement of Behavior Therapy, Los Angeles.

PUTALLAZ, M. (in press). Predicting children's sociometric status from their behavior. *Child Development.*

PUTALLAZ, M., & GOTTMAN, J. (1981). An interactional model of children's entry into peer groups. *Child Development, 52,* 986-994.

PUTALLAZ, M., & GOTTMAN, J. (1983). Social relationship problems in children: An approach to intervention. In B. Lahey & A. Kazdin (Eds.), *Advances in clinical child psychology* (Vol. 6). New York: Plenum Press.

REHM, L. (1977). A self-control model of depression. *Behavior Therapy, 8,* 787-804.

RENSHAW, P., & ASHER, S. R. (in press). Children's goals and strategies for social interaction. *Merrill-Palmer Quarterly.*

ROFF, M., SELLS, S. B., & GOLDEN, M. M. (1972). *Social adjustment and personality development in children.* Minneapolis: University of Minnesota Press.

RUBIN, K. (1982). Social and social-cognitive developmental characteristics of young isolate, normal and sociable children. In K. Rubin & H. Ross (Eds.), *Peer relationships and social skills in childhood.* New York: Springer-Verlag.

SCHWARTZ, R., & GOTTMAN, J. (1976). Toward a task analysis of assertive behavior. *Journal of Consulting and Clinical Psychology, 44,* 910-920.

SHERIF, M., & SHERIF, C. (1964). *Reference groups.* New York: Harper and Row.

SNYDER, M. (1981). Seek, and ye shall find: Testing hypotheses about other people. In T. Higgins, C. Herman, & M. Zanna (Eds.), *Social cognition: The Ontario Symposium.* Hillsdale, NJ: Erlbaum.

STOKES, T., & BAER, D. (1977). An implicit technology of generalization. *Journal of Applied Behavior Analysis, 10,* 345-367.

TEASDALE, J. (1983). Negative thinking in depression: Cause, effect, or reciprocal relationship? In L. Joyce-Moniz, F. Lowe, & P. Higson (Eds.), *Theoretical issues in cognitive-behavioral therapy.* New York: Plenum Press.

TURK, D., MEICHENBAUM, D., & GENEST, M. (1983). *Pain and behavioral medicine.* New York: Guilford Press.

TURK, D., & SPEERS, M. (1983). Cognitive schemata and cognitive processes in cognitive-behavior modification: Going beyond the information given. In P. Kendall (Ed.), *Advances in cognitive-behavioral research and therapy* (Vol. 2). New York: Academic Press.

VAN HASSELT, V., HERSEN, M., WHITEHILL, M., & BELLACK, A. (1979). Social skill assessment and training for children: An evaluative review. *Behaviour Research and Therapy, 17,* 413-437.

WALDROP, M., & HALVERSON, C. (1975). Intensive and extensive peer behavior: Longitudinal and cross-sectional analyses. *Child Development, 46,* 19-26.

WHEELER, V., & LADD, G. (1982). Assessment of children's self-efficacy for social interactions with peers. *Developmental Psychology, 18,* 795-805.

ZAJONC, R. (1980). Feelings and thinking: Preferences need no inferences. *American Psychologist, 35,* 151-175.

Section II
ASSESSMENT AND TREATMENT IN INFANCY, CHILDHOOD, AND ADOLESCENCE

4

Behavior Disorders of Childhood: Diagnosis and Assessment, Taxonomy and Taxometry

THOMAS M. ACHENBACH

CASE EXAMPLE

By way of introduction, consider the following case history:

Nine-year-old Scott M. was brought to a child guidance clinic by his parents. In the initial interview at the clinic, Scott's parents said that they had come at the urging of Scott's third-grade teacher, although they acknowledged that they had long been concerned about the boy, too. Their main concern was that Scott was hyperactive, which is what his teacher had suggested. When asked to describe what they meant, Mrs. M. said that Scott was always doing things he shouldn't. During the preceding week, for example, he had deliberately broken an elaborate Lego structure that his 11-year-old brother had spent several days building. He had also taken his father's power saw, which he had been forbidden to touch. While using the saw, he had cut into a table his father had been refinishing. He often took food from the kitchen, leaving sticky messes of chocolate sauce and honey around the house. When confronted, he usually denied doing these things, even though his involvement was obvious.

Mr. M. said that he had tried to take Scott to sports events, but Scott could not sit still, climbed around on the seats, chattered incessantly, and wanted to have candy, hot dogs, soda, and every souvenir in sight. At home, Scott interfered with other people's television viewing, because he continually talked and made sounds to accompany the action on the screen: "Boom! . . . Bang! . . . Da-da-da!" He also made loud motor sounds and raced about the house pretending to be a motorcycle. Mealtimes were especially hectic, as Scott rejected certain foods with loud complaints of "Yuck!" "Ick!" "Puke!" and vomiting sounds. But he also complained that his brother got more of the foods that he did want. He often got up and walked around while eating, sometimes accompanied by motorcycle sounds.

In the neighborhood, Scott had no playmates because interactions with other children usually ended in fights. Scott occasionally complained about not having friends, but he said it was because certain other kids were out to get him and they kept others from playing with him. Once Scott came home with a bike that he said had been given to him. On another occasion, his mother discovered a baseball glove under some clothes in his bureau drawer. When confronted with it, Scott said he had found it.

Mr. and Mrs. M. could not remember precise details of Scott's developmental history other than that he was born five weeks premature, weighing under five pounds. He seemed to be somewhat slower than his older brother in learning to walk and talk. He was always more active and harder to control than his brother. He had several high fevers during his first year. When asked about convulsions, the M.'s said they weren't sure but he may have had a convulsion once with a fever. Scott did not get along very well with other children in nursery school, but his problems there were not as bad as in elementary school.

In elementary school, Scott's kindergarten teacher said he was immature, but she did not think he should repeat kindergarten. Despite being among the oldest in the class (his birthday was on January 2), Scott was in the lowest reading group in first grade. However, he was promoted to the second-grade class of a teacher who was especially good with slow readers. During second grade, he made slow but definite progress and was not considered a serious behavior problem. In third grade, however, his teacher complained that he was often out of his seat, did not pay attention, talked out of turn, and was not learning. She considered him hyperactive and referred him to the school psychologist for testing. On the WISC-R, he obtained a Verbal IQ of 98, a Performance IQ of 109, and a full-scale IQ of 103. The Peabody

Individual Achievement Test showed that he was more than a year behind his grade placement in most areas. Although Scott sometimes answered impulsively, the psychologist considered the scores to be a reasonable estimate of his ability and achievement.

DIAGNOSIS

Scott is not exactly an unusual case. He may sound familiar. How should we diagnose him?

1) Hyperactive? Or, in the terminology of the current edition of the American Psychiatric Association's (1980) *Diagnostic and Statistical Manual,* Attention Deficit Disorder with Hyperactivity?
2) MBD?
3) Conduct disorder? If so, which of the following drawn from the *Diagnostic and Statistical Manual*?
    (a) Undersocialized Aggressive?
    (b) Undersocialized Nonaggressive?
    (c) Socialized Aggressive?
    (d) Socialized Nonaggressive?
4) Learning disabled?
5) Depressed?
6) Suffering from masked depression?
7) All of the above?
8) None of the above?
9) Does it matter?

Well, whichever alternative we choose, it probably *does* matter. It can affect payments by health insurance and government agencies. It can affect what parents are told and how they view their son and his problems. It can determine who is expected to treat Scott and what type of treatment is used, from stimulant versus antidepressant drugs, to behavior therapy, group therapy, family therapy, or psychotherapy. And it can affect what is done in school, from placement in a special class for emotional disturbance, behavior disorders, or learning disabilities, to a classroom token system or extra attention from Scott's present teacher.

Even if we reject diagnostic labels as meaningless, people carry them around in their heads and use them to organize their thinking about children's problems. In short, diagnostic concepts have consequences.

ASSESSMENT

The behavioral revolution of the 1960s promoted an alternative approach to the diagnosis of behavior disorders, under the banner of *behavioral assessment*. By 1981, Mash and Terdal could compile a hefty tome entitled, *Behavioral Assessment of Children's Disorders*. They cited several contrasts between behavioral assessment and what they called "traditional assessment," meaning mainly psychodynamic, medical, and trait concepts of diagnosis. A fundamental contrast was drawn between the traditional emphasis on inferences about underlying variables—such as psychodynamic constructs, disease entities, and personality—and the behavioral emphasis on observable behaviors and the environmental contingencies supporting them.

The behavioral assessment method par excellence is the structured recording of behaviors observed in natural settings. From the published reports of behavior therapy, we might conclude that structured observations of problem behavior are easy and routine for behavior modifiers. However, Wade, Baker, and Hartmann (1979) found that practicing behavior therapists seldom used trained observers to record problem behavior under natural conditions. In addition to the prohibitive costs and practical obstacles involved in using direct observation for routine clinical assessment, many problem behaviors, such as stealing, firesetting, and fighting, are unlikely to occur under the watchful eyes of trained observers. And even where exceptionally thorough observations have been done in the homes of exceptionally cooperative families, the observed contingencies seem to account for little of the variance in problem behaviors, as Gerald Patterson's (1980) observational tour-de-force illustrates.

Early reports of behavior therapy also suggested that behavioral assessment somehow avoided all the reliability and validity problems of traditional assessment. Yet, in his foreword to Mash and Terdal's book, Patterson (1981) wrote:

> Within a short time, we found ourselves engaged with the traditional psychometric problems of interobserver agreement, validity, stability of behavior over time, bias, the effects of observer presence, and normative data. The old questions are still with us. If anything, they were more demanding and more difficult to answer (p. vii).

To Patterson's list of questions, we could add several more. One is the question of the *representativeness* of any particular sample of behavior with respect to the problems for which a child is referred. Even if observers could avoid affecting the behavior of the child they observe, many problem behaviors are confined to situations in which it would be impossible to place trained observers. Other problem behaviors are of such low frequency that even a large number of observational samples in the appropriate situations would fail to detect them. Consider, for example, the episodes of stealing implied by Scott's parents' report of his coming home with a bicycle that he said had been given him and by their discovery of a baseball glove in his bureau drawer. Or Scott's occasional complaints of lacking friends and blaming kids who were out to get him. Would we be able to obtain direct observational samples representative of these problems?

An additional question might be raised about the power of observational data to indicate the pathognomicity of behavior. If we use orthodox observational methods, we obtain a record of the occurrence of a particular behavior, defined topographically, in a particular situation. However, this record of the actual occurrence of the behavior may be poorly correlated with the malignancy of the behavior in terms of its impact on important people in the child's life, its interference with the child's development, and its prognostic significance.

Scott's destruction of his brother's Lego project and his father's table, as well as the chocolate sauce and honey episodes, would earn low frequency scores on direct observational measures, even if Scott had been undeterred by the presence of an observer. Furthermore, many other nine-year-old boys might commit similar transgressions without falling into the clutches of the mental health system. The pathognomicity of Scott's behavior lay not so much in the intrinsically bizarre or dastardly nature of each deed, but in the *cumulative negative impact* they had on the important people in his life and the apparent *lack of positive interactions* to offset them. In school, the fact that his behavior seemed worse and less tolerable in third grade than second grade could be a function of the expectations of his third-grade teacher, as much as any actual acceleration of his problem behaviors. However, the increasing salience of his failure to meet third-grade standards may have really escalated his problem behaviors.

The limitations of direct observations under natural conditions have spurred some behavior modifiers to advocate what they call *multimethod behavioral assessment* (Nay, 1979). For assessment of children, the multiple methods include interviews, standardized tests, checklists and logbooks completed by parents, observations in natural and clinical settings, and simulation of problem situations. Some of this may sound suspiciously like the "traditional" approaches that were intially rejected by behavior modifiers. Despite the counterrevolutionary flavor of this broadening conception of assessment, however, the initial ideal of behavioral assessment had several salutary effects:

1) It provided a clear-cut *alternative* to the quest for poorly substantiated psychodynamics, diseases, and personality traits.
2) It encouraged mental health workers to *document* the child's actual behavior, instead of concentrating on tenuously inferred constructs.
3) It stimulated examination of the *specific contingencies* affecting the behavior at the present time, instead of looking to the remote past for explanations that were often unverifiable.
4) It emphasized that assessment and intervention should be a *continuous process,* with initial assessment providing a plan for action and subsequent assessments being used to evaluate and modify the interventions.

Nevertheless, even the multimethod behavioral assessment paradigm does not tell us how to *aggregate* data on individual children in order to link them with other children on whom experience has been gained. Without means for linking individuals with others who have similar problems, it is hard to *accumulate* knowledge about the likely causes and most effective interventions for particular kinds of problems. The behavioral assessment paradigm is certainly more neutral and open-ended than traditional diagnostic paradigms, but it cannot escape the need for conceptual categories. For example, how can multimethod behavioral assessment provide a picture of Scott's problems that will apply experience with other children to helping Scott and his family? This is the problem of *taxonomy,* to which we now turn.

TAXONOMY

Taxonomic assumptions are implicit in most approaches to diagnosis and assessment. When we considered possible diagnoses for Scott, we were seeking an appropriate *taxonomic category* for his disorder. Some of the candidates, such as Attention Deficit Disorder, were categories of the DSM-III taxonomy. Others represented categories like those that mental health workers employ with considerable conviction without necessarily equating them with an explicit taxonomy such as the DSM. For example, diagnostic workups are often undertaken to determine whether a child is "depressed," "hyperactive," "learning disabled," "brain damaged," "psychotic," or the like. And case conferences are often enlivened by heated debates over such questions as whether a child is "really" hyperactive or "really" depressed.

It is perhaps ironic that even traditional psychodiagnosis, using projective tests, developmental histories, clinical interviews, IQ tests, and medical data, seldom yields a definite taxonomic decision. Instead of integrating all the different types of diagnostic data into a formal diagnosis, the result is more often a lengthy account of inferred underlying dynamics and determinants. Terms such as depression, brain damage, repressed rage, and ego strength may be woven together without a clear statement of what the disorder in question actually is.

Behavioral assessment is much less explicitly oriented toward disease-like concepts than traditional psychodiagnosis. Nevertheless, it requires some sort of conceptual framework for grouping behaviors or individuals that have something in common. Even though each individual is in many respects unique, we can never develop, validate, or teach differential interventions if we cannot discern the characteristics of children who are more likely to benefit from Intervention A than Intervention B. Similarly, if we wish to find specific etiologies or to plan preventive efforts, we must have a clear picture of what the disorder is whose cause or prevention we seek. We must also be able to distinguish between disorders having different causes and likely to require different kinds of preventive efforts. In short, some kind of taxonomic framework is required if we are to advance our knowledge and apply it to helping individual children. What sort of taxonomic framework should we use?

The DSM-III Nosology

Let us first consider the taxonomic system of the DSM-III, which dominates clinical practice in the United States by virtue of its use for official record-keeping and for third-party payments. Analogous systems, such as the International Classification of Diseases, are used in other countries.

As a formal taxonomy, DSM-III embodies the following advances over the first and second editions of the DSM (American Psychiatric Association, 1952, 1968):

1) The previous mixture of narrative descriptions and inferences has been replaced by explicit criteria for each diagnosis.

2) The criteria for certain adult disorders, such as schizophrenia and major depressions, are based on research diagnostic criteria (RDC) evolved from efforts to make reliable discriminations between disorders.

3) Unsubstantiated inferences about psychodynamic mechanisms have been dropped.

4) The scope of diagnosis has been broadened by adding axes for non-psychiatric medical conditions, severity of psychosocial stressors, and level of adaptive functioning.

Despite advances in the formal properties of the DSM taxonomy, these advances may not have contributed much to the classification of children's disorders. There were no research diagnostic criteria on which to base the DSM criteria for children's disorders. Instead, the criteria for the DSM-III children's disorders originated in the DSM committee, with little basis in research.

Furthermore, unlike adult disorders, DSM-III diagnoses of children's disorders require other people's reports of behavior that the clinician is unlikely to observe. In the diagnosis of Attention Deficit Disorder, for example, the DSM specifies that "the signs must be reported by adults in the child's environment, such as parents and teachers" (American Psychiatric Association, 1980, p. 43). Similarly, in the conduct disorders, the clinician is unlikely to observe and the child is unlikely to report the requisite behaviors, such as physical violence, theft, and lying.

The clinician must not only obtain the basic data from others, but also judge whether the reported behavior deviates sufficiently from norms for the child's peers to meet the diagnostic criteria. To qualify for the diagnosis of Attention Deficit Disorder, for example, the DSM states that "the child displays, for his or her mental and chronological age, signs of developmentally inappropriate inattention, impulsivity, and hyperactivity" (p. 43). Yet, no operations are specified for either obtaining behavioral reports from parents and teachers or for judging whether the reported behavior is sufficiently inappropriate for the child's age to meet the diagnostic criteria. Furthermore, the judgment of each criterion must be made in a yes-or-no fashion, despite the fact that the criterial behaviors are specified in quasi-quantitative terms. The behavioral criteria for Attention Deficit Disorder, for example, include the following:

- "*Often* doesn't seem to listen."
- "*Easily* distracted."
- "Shifts *excessively* from one activity to another."
- "*Frequently* calls out in class."

How "often," "easily," "excessively," and "frequently" must the behavior occur to meet each of these criteria?

Once a yes-or-no judgment is made about each of these criteria, the number of "yes" judgments must be counted to determine whether they reach the criteria of three symptoms of *inattention*, three of *impulsivity*, and two of *hyperactivity*. Children for whom a "yes" judgment has been made on the requisite number of criteria are then concluded to belong to the category of those who have the disorder, whereas children falling short of the requisite number are excluded from the category. Children who are very extreme on all the behavioral criteria are categorized with those who meet only the minimum number of criteria required for the diagnosis. Likewise, children whose behavior also meets the criteria for several other diagnoses are categorized with children whose behavior meets the criteria for no other diagnoses or a different set of diagnoses. The final yes-or-no diagnosis thus camouflages the *quantitative variation* in specific behaviors, the *number* of behavioral criteria that are met to make the diagnosis, and the child's *overall pattern* of behavior.

Consider Scott as an example. Based on reports by Scott's parents and teacher, a clinician could conclude that Scott easily meets all the DSM criteria for Attention Deficit Disorder with Hyperactivity. However, he would also meet the criteria for Undersocialized, Nonaggressive Conduct Disorder; Developmental Reading Disorder; Developmental Arithmetic Disorder; and possibly Schizoid Disorder of Childhood. Do any of these categorical diagnoses, or all of them together, capture important characteristics that Scott shares with other clinically referred nine-year-old boys who might profit from similar interventions? This question would, of course, require long-term, programmatic research to answer.

We already have evidence, however, that the efforts to make the DSM more reliable via a set of fixed rules for each diagnostic category have not succeeded for children's disorders. Appendix F of the DSM reports reliability coefficients for diagnostic agreements between pairs of clinicians in field trials using an early draft of DSM-III and then a later draft. Although reliability improved from the early draft to the later draft for diagnoses of adults, it worsened for diagnoses of children.

This was true not only for the Axis I psychiatric syndromes, but also for the other three axes assessed: Axis II, Personality Disorders and Specific Developmental Disorders; Axis IV, Severity of Psychosocial Stressors; and Axis V, Highest Level of Adaptive Functioning Past Year. Thus, the changes that improved the reliability of adult diagnoses seem to have *reduced* the reliability of child diagnoses.

Furthermore, two studies have shown worse reliability for DSM-III diagnoses of standardized case histories than for DSM-II diagnoses, which were themselves not very reliable (Mattison, Cantwell, Russell, & Will, 1979; Mezzich & Mezzich, 1979). DSM-III's explicitly categorical nosology, using fixed decision rules to assign cases to categories in a yes-or-no fashion, thus leaves much to be desired as a taxonomy of children's disorders.

Other Nosological Taxonomies

All three editions of the DSM have been shaped largely by the needs of adult psychiatric practice. Two nosological systems have been proposed for children's disorders.

The neglect of children in the first edition of the DSM (American Psychiatric Association, 1952) prompted the Committee on Child Psychiatry of the Group for the Advancement of Psychiatry (GAP, 1966) to formulate an alternative system for children's disorders. Although the GAP Committee followed the traditional practice of starting with their own clinical concepts of disorders, they tried to incorporate developmental considerations more than the DSM has. For example, they included a category of *healthy responses* to encompass normal reactions to developmental crises, such as the separation anxiety shown by six-month-old babies, preschoolers' phobias, adolescent identity crises, and grief reactions to the death of loved ones.

The GAP committee held that its definitions of disorders were as operational as possible. Some categories were highly inferential, however, as exemplified by the definition of Psychoneurotic Disorders as

> . . . disorders based on unconscious conflicts over the handling of sexual and aggressive impulses which, though removed from awareness by the mechanism of repression, remain active and unresolved. . . . The anxiety, acting as a danger signal to the ego, ordinarily sets into operation certain defense mechanisms, in addition to repression, and leads to the formation of psychological

symptoms which symbolically deal with the conflict, thus achieving a partial though unhealthy solution. (GAP, 1966, pp. 229-230)

No explicit criteria, rules, or assessment operations were provided for making diagnoses. Therefore, it should not be surprising that, despite being designed specifically for childhood disorders, the GAP system's reliability has been found to be no better than that of the DSM (Beitchman, Dielman, Landis, Benson, & Kemp, 1978; Freeman, 1971).

Another nosological taxonomy for childhood disorders was drafted by the World Health Organization (Rutter, Shaffer, & Shepherd, 1975). Like DSM-III, it is multiaxial. However, its axes are *psychiatric syndromes; level of intellectual functioning; biological factors;* and *psychological and social factors.* Interjudge reliability for five broad diagnostic categories of the WHO system has been found to be somewhat better than similar reliability for GAP and DSM-III childhood diagnoses (Rutter et al., 1975).

By using a separate axis for level of intellectual functioning, the WHO system avoids making mental retardation a category on the same axis as psychiatric syndromes. As Rutter and Shaffer (1980) have pointed out, the WHO approach of separating intellectual functioning from psychiatric syndromes avoids problems arising from DSM-III's inclusion of mental retardation as an Axis I category. For example, DSM-III states that certain diagnoses, such as attention deficit disorders, should not be made if the condition is "due to mental retardation." This implies that retardation per se can cause attention deficit disorders. Yet many retarded children would not meet the criteria for attention deficit disorders, though some would. If a retarded child shows the behavior problems imputed to attention deficit disorders, should we dismiss these problems because the child is retarded?

The point is that retardation is operationally defined in terms of IQ test scores, which reflect *quantitative* deviance from performance on a particular set of tasks by normative samples of a child's agemates. A low score on the cognitive dimension assessed by the IQ test is not automatically equivalent to any particular syndrome, disorder, or categorical entity, and does not necessarily account for any particular behavioral syndrome. It may make sense to establish cutoff points on the IQ dimension to discriminate between children whose educational needs differ, such as those with IQs below 50, 50 to 75, and above 75. However, a particular score on the dimension does not intrinsically represent a psychiatric disorder; such a score may be accompanied by any of a variety of behavior problems, as well as by no serious behavior problems.

In Scott's case, his IQ of 103 rules out a diagnosis of mental retardation, but his poor school performance qualifies him for DSM diagnoses of Developmental Reading Disorder and Developmental Arithmetic Disorder. His poor school performance is certainly cause for concern, but it is not necessarily a categorical entity any more than a low IQ score would be. Instead, it represents a *level* of accomplishment that falls below the norms for his age. As the WHO taxonomy illustrates, a low level of functioning on a particular dimension need not be equated with a categorical disorder (Rutter et al., 1975).

Multivariate Approaches to Taxonomy

The lack of satisfactory diagnostic categories for child psychopathology has prompted numerous efforts to identify syndromes empirically through statistical analyses of associations among reported behaviors. One of the earliest of these efforts was carried out in the 1930s by Ackerson (1942), who computed correlations between all possible pairs of 125 behavior problems scored from child guidance case histories. Jenkins and Glickman (1946) then derived syndromes from this mass of correlations by picking out pairs of highly correlated items and adding items that correlated with each member of the highly correlated pairs. They used a combination of statistical criteria and clinical judgment to decide when to stop adding items.

A similar study by Hewitt and Jenkins (1946) and later reanalyses of the same data yielded syndromes that became widely cited in the child clinical literature, such as the Unsocialized Aggressive and Socialized Delinquent. These syndromes ultimately served as prototypes for some of the DSM-II categories of childhood disorders, such as the Unsocialized Aggressive Reaction of Childhood and the Group Delinquent Reaction of Childhood. However, the initial research data were secondhand reports in case histories, the derivation of syndromes from correlations was largely subjective, and no operational definitions were provided that could be applied to new cases for either clinical or research purposes. Furthermore, when the DSM-II committee incorporated the results of this work, they did so by describing their own clinical concepts of the disorders.

As electronic computers and multivariate statistics became available, there were increasing efforts to derive syndromes through factor analysis of data from parents, teachers, mental health workers, and case histories. Despite the diversity of informants, rating scales, subject populations, and statistical methods, there was considerable convergence in the identification of a few broad-band syndromes and more numerous narrow-band syndromes (Achenbach & Edelbrock, 1978; Quay, 1979). In almost all studies where the methodology permitted identification of broad-band syndromes, one syndrome comprising inhibited, fearful, overcontrolled behavior and a second syndrome comprising aggressive, impulsive, undercontrolled behavior were found. This dichotomy was variously designated as "overinhibited versus aggressive," "personality disorder versus conduct disorder," and "internalizing versus externalizing."

Among studies where the methodology permitted identification of more differentiated, narrow-band syndromes, at least six studies produced syndromes that could be labeled as aggressive, delinquent, hyperactive, anxious, schizoid, depressed, social withdrawal, and somatic complaints (see Achenbach & Edelbrock, 1978). Additional syndromes, designated as sexual problems, immature, obsessive-compulsive, uncommunicative, academic disability, and sleep problems, were also found in three or four studies.

Despite the apparent progress in statistically deriving syndromes, little was done to provide operational procedures for grouping children according to the syndromes they manifested. Instead, most efforts ended with the coining of names for the statistically derived syndromes, plus some hopeful speculation on what the children are like who manifest each syndrome.

Unfortunately, the statistically derived syndromes reveal only the associations among items and not necessarily the *patterns* of behavior that distinguish individual children from one another. Furthermore, the statistical associations among items typically reflect the perspectives of one type of informant, such as a parent or teacher. Different informants are involved in very different types of interaction with children and have different standards for judging them. Whose view of the child should we believe?

An additional weakness of most of the multivariate efforts stems from the haphazardness of their samples, in which children of both sexes and diverse ages were mixed in varying proportions. The repeated identification of certain syndromes across samples varying in composition implies that these syndromes are robust. Yet, analyses of samples containing children of both sexes and diverse ages can obscure syndromes that are peculiar to one sex or a particular developmental period. Moreover, the differing base rates and implications of particular behaviors for boys versus girls and children of different ages undermine the clinical utility of syndromes derived from samples combining both sexes and diverse ages. Fear of school, for example, may be associated with an empirically derived syndrome. Yet, it may be wrong to ascribe the same clinical significance to it in six-year-olds as in 14-year-olds. Likewise, a particular behavior may have positive statistical associations with several other behaviors at one age, but negative associations with these same behaviors at a later age. Analyses of samples containing both these age groups would fail to reveal any statistical relations among the behaviors, thereby obscuring the associations that in fact exist, but are of opposite sign at different ages.

Many of the weaknesses of the multivariate studies are not inherent in the approach. Instead, they result from the subordination of multivariate statistical techniques to a categorical conceptual paradigm. Thus, while the lack of diagnostic categories for child psychopathology is what instigated the empirical search for syndromes, multivariate statistics were seen largely as a tool for discovering entities analogous to those of traditional diagnostic classifications. An example is the grouping of characteristics that Jenkins originally called the Unsocialized Aggressive Child and that has been approximated in several factor-analytic studies. When it was incorporated into the DSM-II, it was defined as follows:

> This disorder is characterized by overt or covert hostile disobedience, quarrelsomeness, physical and verbal aggressiveness, vengefulness, and destructiveness. Temper tantrums, solitary stealing, lying, and hostile teasing of other children are common. These patients usually have no consistent parental acceptance and discipline. This diagnosis should be distinguished from *Antisocial personality, Runaway reaction of childhood,* and *Group delinquent reaction of childhood.* (American Psychiatric Association, 1968, p. 51)

Despite the admonition to distinguish this disorder from certain other disorders, no criteria were provided for determining that the disorder was actually present or for ruling out the other disorders. The DSM-III's version of it, the Undersocialized Aggressive Conduct Disorder, has more explicit criteria but is distinguished from other disorders mainly by the statement that "if 18 or older, does not meet the criteria for Antisocial Personality Disorder" (American Psychiatric Association, 1980, p. 48). What began as a set of quantitative relations among behavior ratings has thus become an entity to be categorically distinguished from other entities, however imperfectly.

When multivariate findings are cast into the mold of a categorical taxonomy, many of the advantages of the multivariate approach are lost. Full utilization of the power of quantitative methods requires a conceptual paradigm different from that of categorical taxonomies. We will now consider a conceptual paradigm for more explicitly capitalizing on the power of quantitative methods to express relations among large numbers of variables.

TAXOMETRY

The term *taxometry* has been used in several senses. It has been used to refer specifically to cluster analysis as a quantitative method for creating taxonomies (Sokol & Sneath, 1963). Paul Meehl has recently used it in reference to psychometric procedures for discriminating between individuals who have a particular type of disorder, especially schizophrenia, and those who do not have the disorder. More broadly, Meehl calls taxometrics "the branch of applied mathematics that treats problems of classification" (Meehl & Golden, 1982, p. 127). Meehl maintains that "the purpose of taxometrics is to help the investigator identify and sort those categories of individuals that are in some sense 'really in nature' " (p. 127). He provides an impressive set of arguments for the centrality of taxonomic problems in research on psychopathology, and he offers some high-powered mathematical approaches to solving them. He also implies that *types* rather than *dimensions* are the proper focus of taxometrics. Indeed, he may be correct vis-à-vis adult schizophrenia, which is the main focus of his taxometric efforts.

However, one need not be wedded to the notion of categorical types nor need one master Meehl's esoteric formulations to see the possible benefits of a metrical framework for both the assessment and conceptualization of behavior disorders of childhood. Instead, taxometric approaches can contribute to our understanding of child psychopathology in a number of ways.

Aggregation of Molecular Data

One contribution is in the aggregation of molecular assessment data into more molar conceptual units, as follows:

1) Most of the behavior problems for which help is sought differ only *quantitatively* from the behavior of children who are not considered

to need special help. In Scott's case, for example, there was no single behavior or incident that was so intrinsically pathognomonic as to instigate referral by itself. Instead, referral was the outcome of a long-term accumulation of problem behaviors, combined with lagging social and academic skills. This does not necessarily mean that all children's behavior problems can be viewed as quantitative variations on normal functioning. The very early and pervasive deviance of autistic children, for example, may not represent quantitative variants of normal behavior. A few children who show precipitous changes from attained levels of functioning, such as psychotic breaks, may also be exceptions, although knowledge of their characteristic functioning on age-appropriate dimensions may nevertheless be helpful in setting goals for intervention.

2) The classic scenario for the identification of syndromes has starred astute clinicians who brilliantly detect the co-occurrence of certain anomalous characteristics. Examples include the identification of mongolism (or Down's syndrome) by Langdon Down in 1866; the identification of phenylketonuria (or Fölling's disease) by Fölling in 1934; and the identification of infantile autism (or Kanner's syndrome) by Leo Kanner in 1943. However, the diversity of problem behaviors, complicated further by the *variability* of each child's behavior, poses a much more massive information-processing task than the detection of blatant anomalies. Since relevant behaviors may not be observed by the clinician, standardized reports and multivariate statistics are needed to sift through, aggregate, and reduce large quantities of data.

3) Since interventions seldom succeed in replacing each problem behavior with a socially desirable behavior, assessment of *change* requires quantitative indices of aggregates of behaviors targeted for reduction and those targeted for strengthening.

Providing a Normative-Developmental Context

A second way in which a taxometric paradigm can contribute is by providing a normative-developmental context in which to judge the behavior of particular children. By normative-developmental, I mean merely the construction of norms for each age by obtaining standardized data on representative samples of children, in the same way as is done for IQ and achievement tests. Although certain developmental theories may help us understand the progress of adaptive development, one need not espouse developmental theories to recognize that behavioral problems and competencies typically change with age, much as height, weight, cognitive functioning, and school achievement do. Some specific implications are as follows:

1) Aggregates of behavioral problems and competencies derived via multivariate statistics constitute quantitative composite variables which can be scaled according to distributions of scores for normative samples of a particular age.
2) Because both the patterning and prevalence of particular behaviors change with age, separate multivariate analyses should be performed on children of different ages. The aggregates thus obtained can be scored in terms of normative distributions for each of the relevant ages. This makes it possible to reflect age changes in the patterning as well as the distribution of behaviors.
3) By computing norm-based standard scores for a child's reported behaviors, we can determine the degree to which the child's reported behaviors deviate from those reported for peers. Displaying scales in a profile format makes it possible to visually compare the relative deviance in each area.
4) As a child grows older, we can continue to assess the degree of deviance by reference to norms for each successive age.

Forming Typologies

A third type of contribution offered by the taxometric paradigm is in the grouping of children according to their overall patterns on the quantitatively derived aggregates of reported behaviors, as exemplified in the following ways:

1) We can use quantitative algorithms, such as cluster analysis, to group children according to similarities in their profile patterns.
2) Once profile types have been identified, we can compute correlations between a child's profile and each profile type to determine the *degree* of his or her similarity to each type, rather than having to assign the child to a category in an all-or-none fashion.
3) When investigating correlates of profile types, we can determine how strongly children's profiles must resemble a type for the children to share the correlates of the type.

Coordinating Multiple Perspectives on Behavior

Viewing assessment and taxonomy from a metrical perspective highlights another issue that is equally important for nonmetrical approaches, as well. This is the fact that there is no absolute criterion for what a behavior disorder "really" is. The judgment that help is needed for a child's behavior is always a function of many variables, including the situations in which particular behavior occurs, the people with whom the child is interacting, their impact on the child, and the subjective standards of those who evaluate the child's behavior. In short, behavior disorders do not exist "out there," independent of anybody's perceptions and judgments.

Family systems therapists argue that a child referred for help is a symptom of a troubled family and that we should therefore focus on the family system, rather than the child. They are certainly correct in holding that the problems do not inhere exclusively in the child and that family dynamics help to determine who is singled out as having problems. However, the family is not the only relevant system; troubled children are often also identified as having problems by other systems, such as the school and peer group. In most cases, helping the child indeed requires changes in the family, but there is little evidence that family therapy automatically improves the child's functioning in the nonfamily systems, especially if the child has a long history of problems outside the family context.

Recognition of the relativism involved in evaluating behavior problems does not necessarily dictate any particular therapeutic approach, such as family therapy. Instead, it underlines the fact that all assessment approaches impose an epistemological framework on the phenomena of interest—that is, each approach defines the phenomena in a particular way that highlights certain features but shuts out other features. When we use trained observers, the data they obtain are shaped and limited by the procedures and situations they employ and by their impact on the subject's behavior. The same is true for reports by parents, teachers, clinicians, and children themselves. Although this is acknowledged by most approaches to assessment, there nevertheless seems to be an implicit conviction that children's behavior disorders have a reality independent of any particular situation and observer. Consequently, poor agreement between a parent and teacher, for example, is often used to cast doubt on the "reliability" of one of the informants. In nosologies such as the DSM, it is the clinician who, despite not observing many of the criterial behaviors, must ultimately decide whether Scott really has an attention deficit disorder, conduct disorder, etc.

Yet, if we take a metrical approach seriously, it is clear that several measurement systems may validly convey different pictures of a child.

Each of the pictures may need to be understood in its own right, without necessarily being rejected because it disagrees with others. As emphasized by Heisenberg's Uncertainty Principle in particle physics, our knowledge is always a function of a particular assessment system which inevitably interacts with the phenomena being assessed. And, because all assessments of children's behavior depend on human judgments of the behavior, we must be aware, as exquisitely dramatized in the Japanese film *Roshomon,* that the truth depends on who is telling it. The different pictures of children seen by parents, teachers, observers, and the children themselves may each contain very different but important truths. To test the value of data from each source, we need to make these pictures as clear and distinct as possible.

SOME ILLUSTRATIONS

I will close by illustrating some aspects of a taxometric approach in more concrete form, as applied to Scott, who was described earlier in the narrative fashion of the traditional case history.

The Child Behavior Checklist

In addition to the usual intake interview from which the narrative description was derived, Scott's parents each filled out the Child Behavior Checklist (Achenbach, 1978; Achenbach & Edelbrock, 1983). This is a questionnaire designed to obtain parents' descriptions of their children's behavioral problems and competencies in a standardized format. Parents can fill it out in about 15 minutes at home or in the waiting room prior to their first interview.

Total Social Competence and Behavior Problem Scores

The parents' reports of the quantity and quality of their child's participation in activities, social relationships, and school yields a total social competence score, while their ratings of 118 behavior problem items yields a total behavior problem score. In a home interview survey of 1,300 parents of randomly selected children not referred for mental health services, we obtained normative distributions of social competence and behavior problem scores for each sex at ages four through 16 (Achenbach & Edelbrock, 1981). We then experimented with ways to use the social competence and behavior problem scores to discriminate between the nonreferred children and 1,300 children who had been referred for outpatient mental health services. We found that most of the clinically referred children had social competence scores that were below the 10th percentile of the nonreferred children's scores and behavior problem scores that were above the 90th percentile of nonreferred children's scores. Using these scores as cutoff points generally proved superior to fancier statistical procedures for discriminating between children who were in the normal versus clinical range (see Achenbach & Edelbrock, 1983, for details).

In Scott's case, the total social competence score obtained from his mother's Child Behavior Checklist was 8, and from his father's Checklist was 7. These are both well *below* the score of 16 that constitutes the 10th percentile of social competence scores for our normative sample of boys of Scott's age.

Scott's total behavior problem scores were 77 on his mother's Checklist and 73 on his father's Checklist. Both of these are well *above* the score of 40 that represents the 90th percentile for our normative sample.

Not only are Scott's scores beyond the cutoff points, but their magnitude is also quite typical of the scores obtained by boys referred to outpatient mental health services. Thus, our normative-developmental framework for judging the competencies and problems reported by Scott's parents places him at a point on a continuum of competencies and problems that is clearly deviant from his normal agemates but that is not much more deviant than many other boys referred for outpatient services. His parents' reports indicate definite cause for concern, not only in terms of their referral complaints of "hyperactivity" and "doing things he shouldn't," but also in terms of many other aspects of his behavior.

Scale Scores of the Child Behavior Profile

Moving from the global level of total scores, we can also view Scott's reported behaviors in terms of more differentiated dimensions of competencies and problems. This is done by considering Scott's scores on the Child Behavior Profile, which is scored from the Child Behavior Checklist. Figure 1 shows the three social competence scales scored from Scott's mother's and father's Checklists. The distributions of scores reflect those found in our normative samples. According to his mother's report, Scott's participation and skill in activities is in the low normal range, whereas his social and school functioning are below the second percentile of our normative samples. Mr. M.'s ratings place Scott slightly lower in the normal range on the Activities scale, but at the same points as Mrs. M.'s ratings on the Social and School scales. Thus, it appears that Scott's most severe deficits are in the social and school areas, although his involvement in activities is also at the low end of the normal range.

As for behavior problems, we have derived syndromes empirically by factor analyzing the behavior problems reported for clinically referred children of each sex within different age ranges. Figure 2 shows behavior problem scales based on the nine syndromes that we empirically identified for six- to 11-year-old boys. The distribution of scores for each scale reflects the distribution found in our normative samples of nonreferred boys. The Profile drawn with a solid line shows how the behavior problems reported by Scott's mother compare with those reported for nonreferred six- to 11-year-old boys. As you can see, Scott is indeed reported to be deviant on the scale that we call Hyperactive.

Scott is even more deviant, however, on the Aggressive and Social Withdrawal scales, and nearly as deviant on the Depressed and Delinquent scales. Thus, even though Scott's mother does report behavior problems involving hyperactivity, the term "hyperactivity" fails to capture the full extent or patterning of Scott's reported deviance from a normative sample of his agemates. According to the profile, it is misleading to view Scott as merely a hyperactive child. Although Scott's parents had mentioned some of the aggressive and delinquent behavior indicated on Scales VIII and IX, the extent of deviance in these areas and in areas indicated by the Depressed and Social Withdrawal scales was not evident from the interview.

The Checklist filled out by Mr. M. indicated slightly fewer problems (a total score of 73 versus 77 on Mrs. M.'s Checklist), but both Checklists yielded similar overall Profile patterns. Upon questioning by the therapist, it became clear that the slightly lower score on the Aggressive scale scored from Mr. M.'s Checklist mainly reflected the greater intensity of certain behaviors (such as arguing, disobedience, and screaming) in the presence of Mrs. M. than Mr. M.

Profile Pattern

So far, I have been discussing the Child Behavior Checklist and Profile as means for obtaining standardized, quantifiable *descriptions* of behavior, *aggregating* the behavior in terms of scales, and *comparing* a child's standing on each scale with that of normative samples of

REVISED CHILD BEHAVIOR PROFILE
Social Competence—Boys Aged 4-5, 6-11, 12-16

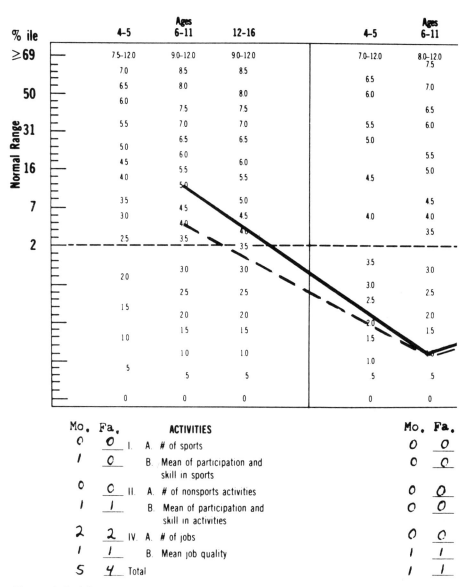

FIGURE 1. Social competence scores derived from Child Behavior Checklists filled out by Scott's mother and father. Copyright 1982, T. M. Achenbach.

REVISED CHILD BEHAVIOR PROFILE
Social Competence—Boys Aged 4-5, 6-11, 12-16

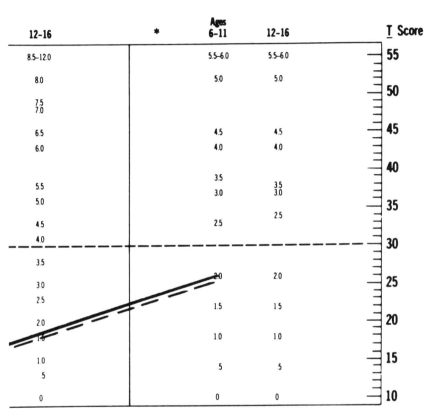

	SOCIAL	Mo.	Fa.		SCHOOL
III.	A. # of organizations	O	O	VII. 1.	Mean performance
	B. Mean of participation in organizations	I	I	2.	Special class
V.	1. # of friends	I	I	3.	Repeated grade
	2. Frequency of contacts with friends	O	O	4.	School problems
VI.	A. Behavior with others	2	2	Total	
	B. Behavior alone				

*Not scored for 4-5-year-olds

Total

Mother ——
Father — — —

REVISED CHILD BEHAVIOR PROFILE
Behavior Problems—Boys Aged 6-11

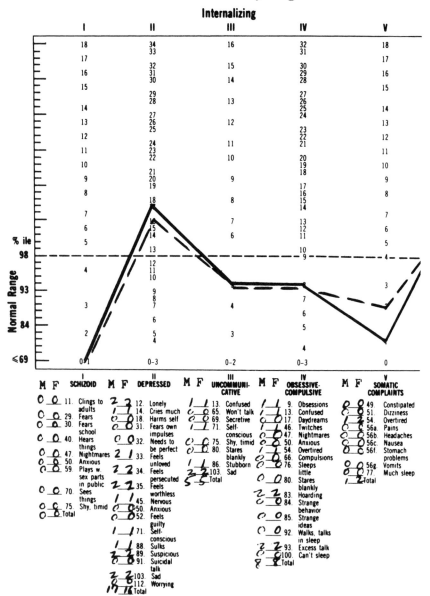

FIGURE 2. Behavior problem scores derived from Child Behavior Checklists filled out by Scott's mother and father. Copyright 1982, T. M. Achenbach.

REVISED CHILD BEHAVIOR PROFILE
Behavior Problems—Boys Aged 6-11

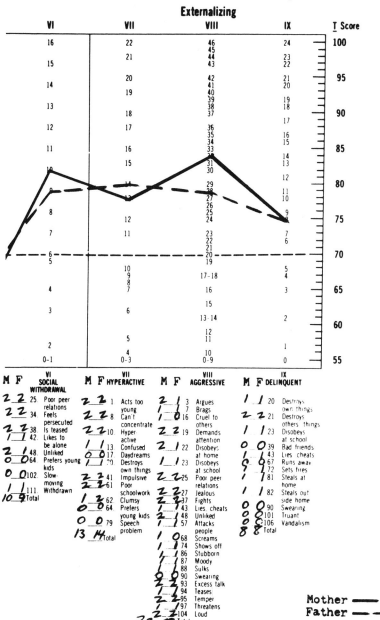

agemates. This enables us to see where the child's problems and competencies are concentrated, as perceived by his or her parents, in comparison with parental reports of the behavior of nonreferred children. However, we also need to *group* children according to similarities that will help us apply previously accumulated knowledge to each new case.

We have cluster analyzed profiles in order to form groups of children whose patterns of parent-reported behavior are similar. Unlike classification of profiles in a categorical fashion, as is done with MMPI high point codes, our cluster analyses use quantitative criteria to group profiles according to the degree of similarity between their entire patterns. Exceptionally low scores on some scales can thus be as influential in determining certain profile types as exceptionally high scores.

Each cluster of similar profiles in our cluster analysis is operationally defined by a particular set of standard scores on the scales of the profile. This means that we can compute a correlation between a child's profile and each of the types in order to quantify the similarity of the child's reported behavior to that of each previously identified group. We use the one-way intraclass correlation to compute the similarity of a child's profile to each type (Achenbach & Edelbrock, 1983; Edelbrock & Achenbach, 1980). A computer-scored version of the Child Behavior Profile automatically computes and prints out the correlation between a child's profile and each of the types for his or her age and sex. Scott's profile correlated highest with a type that has its highest points on the Depressed, Social Withdrawal, and Aggressive scales. Although we have also identified a profile type that is elevated mainly on the Hyperactive scale, Scott's deviance on this scale did not exceed that of most other clinically referred boys sufficiently to earn a large correlation with the Hyperactive profile type.

Scott's intraclass correlation with the Depressed-Social Withdrawal-Aggressive type was .41. This may not sound high, but the intraclass correlation follows a different metric than the more familiar Pearson correlation. The equivalent Pearson correlation would be about .76. Scott thus appears fairly similar to a particular group of boys previously identified in our cluster analyses of clinically referred children.

We are currently studying children whose profiles correlate well with the types we have identified. We have some evidence that boys having the Depressed-Social Withdrawal-Aggressive pattern generally show worse outcomes after typical mental health services than boys having most other profile patterns. They are therefore a group for which we probably have to devise some new interventions.

The Teacher's Report Form

I previously stressed the need for viewing children's behavior from multiple perspectives. The profiles in Figures 1 and 2 illustrated two slightly different perspectives, those of Scott's mother and father. In this case, they did not differ much, although sometimes the profile scores from a mother's and father's Checklists do differ in important ways. When they do differ, this should not be written off as unreliability or error. Instead, the discrepancies may be clinically informative. They should be investigated to determine whether they reflect disagreements in judging particular behavior, differences in opportunities to observe the behavior or in parents' effects on the occurrence of the behavior, or quirks of the parents that deserve special attention.

Next to parents, teachers are often the second most important adult judges of children's behavior. In Scott's case it was his teacher who actually instigated the clinical referral. To obtain teachers' perspectives, we have developed a companion questionnaire called the Teacher's Report Form of the Child Behavior Checklist (Achenbach & Edelbrock, 1983; Edelbrock & Achenbach, 1984). It has many of the same behavior problems as the parent form, but replaces items that teachers would not observe with items that they are more likely to observe. For example, items such as Disobedient at home, Nightmares, Steals at home, and Wets the bed are replaced with items such as Difficulty following directions, Overconforms to rules, Disturbs other pupils, and Hums or makes odd noises in class.

The parents' reports of their child's involvement in activities and social relationships are replaced with teachers' ratings on four general adaptive characteristics that discriminate well between referred and nonreferred children. These are: How hard the child is working; how appropriately the child is behaving; how much the child is learning; and how happy the child is. The teacher is also asked to rate the child's performance in each academic subject and to provide a variety of clinically useful information.

The Teacher Profile

The teacher's ratings are scored on the Teacher Version of the Child Behavior Profile. Normative data were obtained by having teachers fill out the Teacher's Report on randomly selected, nonreferred children. Behavior problem scales were derived by factor analyzing teach-

THE CHILD BEHAVIOR PROFILE—TEACHER'S REPORT VERSION
Teacher-Reported Adaptive Functioning— Boys Aged 6-11

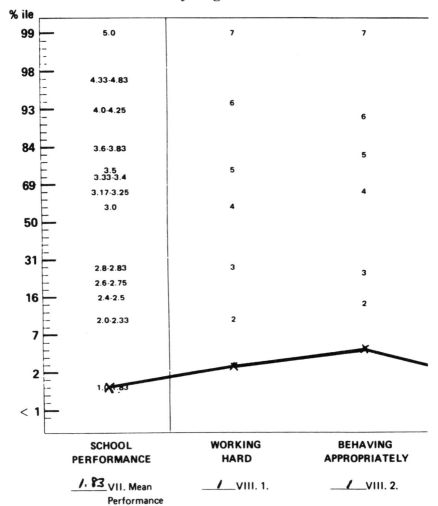

FIGURE 3. Ratings of academic performance and adaptive characteristics by Scott's teacher. Copyright 1982, C. S. Edelbrock & T. M. Achenbach.

THE CHILD BEHAVIOR PROFILE—TEACHER'S REPORT VERSION
Teacher-Reported Adaptive Functioning— Boys Aged 6-11

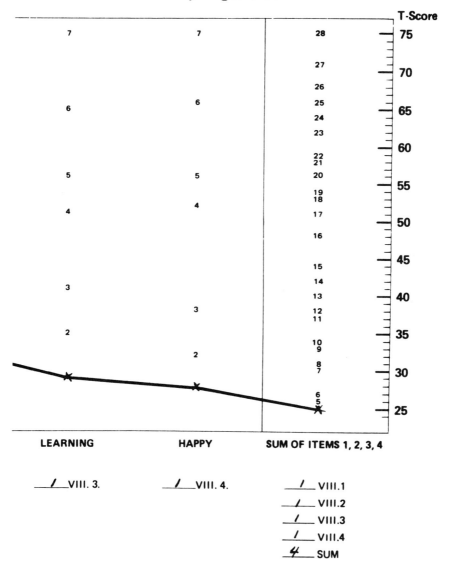

__/__VIII. 3.	__/__VIII. 4.	__/__ VIII.1
		__/__ VIII.2
		__/__ VIII.3
		__/__ VIII.4
		__4__ SUM

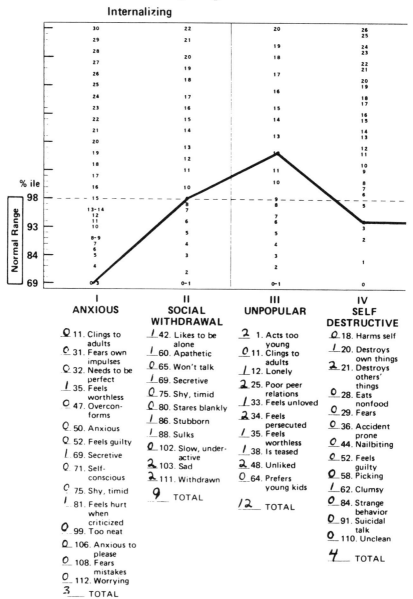

FIGURE 4. Ratings of behavior problems by Scott's teacher. Copyright 1982, C. S. Edelbrock & T. M. Achenbach.

TEACHER REPORTED BEHAVIOR PROBLEMS
Boys Aged 6-11

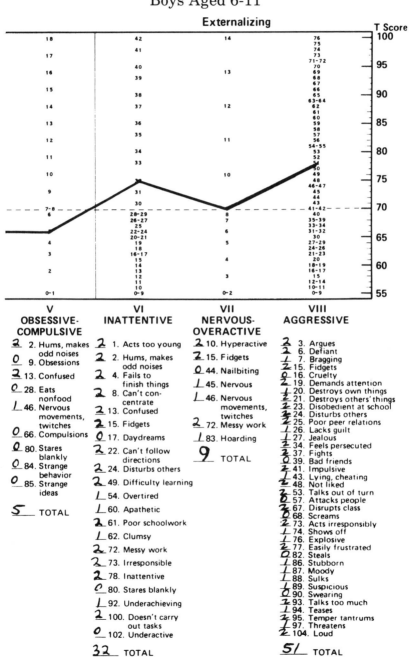

Externalizing

T Score

V	VI	VII	VIII
OBSESSIVE-COMPULSIVE	**INATTENTIVE**	**NERVOUS-OVERACTIVE**	**AGGRESSIVE**

V OBSESSIVE-COMPULSIVE

2 2. Hums, makes odd noises
0 9. Obsessions
2 13. Confused
0 28. Eats nonfood
1 46. Nervous movements, twitches
0 66. Compulsions
0 80. Stares blankly
0 84. Strange behavior
0 85. Strange ideas

5 TOTAL

VI INATTENTIVE

2 1. Acts too young
2 2. Hums, makes odd noises
2 4. Fails to finish things
2 8. Can't concentrate
2 13. Confused
2 15. Fidgets
0 17. Daydreams
2 22. Can't follow directions
2 24. Disturbs others
2 49. Difficulty learning
1 54. Overtired
1 60. Apathetic
2 61. Poor schoolwork
1 62. Clumsy
2 72. Messy work
2 73. Irresponsible
2 78. Inattentive
0 80. Stares blankly
1 92. Underachieving
2 100. Doesn't carry out tasks
0 102. Underactive

32 TOTAL

VII NERVOUS-OVERACTIVE

2 10. Hyperactive
2 15. Fidgets
0 44. Nailbiting
1 45. Nervous
1 46. Nervous movements, twitches
2 72. Messy work
1 83. Hoarding

9 TOTAL

VIII AGGRESSIVE

2 3. Argues
2 6. Defiant
1 7. Bragging
2 15. Fidgets
0 16. Cruelty
2 19. Demands attention
1 20. Destroys own things
2 21. Destroys others' things
2 23. Disobedient at school
4 24. Disturbs others
2 25. Poor peer relations
1 26. Lacks guilt
1 27. Jealous
2 34. Feels persecuted
2 37. Fights
0 39. Bad friends
2 41. Impulsive
2 43. Lying, cheating
2 48. Not liked
2 53. Talks out of turn
0 57. Attacks people
2 67. Disrupts class
0 68. Screams
2 73. Acts irresponsibly
1 74. Shows off
1 76. Explosive
2 77. Easily frustrated
0 82. Steals
1 86. Stubborn
1 87. Moody
1 88. Sulks
1 89. Suspicious
0 90. Swearing
2 93. Talks too much
1 94. Teases
2 95. Temper tantrums
1 97. Threatens
2 104. Loud

51 TOTAL

ers' ratings of the behavior problems of clinically referred children. Figure 3 shows Scott's teacher's ratings of his academic performance, the four adaptive characteristics, and a composite of the four adaptive characteristics. On all these indices, Scott received the lowest possible scores, comparable to approximately the lowest 2% of our normative samples.

Figure 4 shows the profile of Scott's teacher's ratings of his behavior problems. Note that the scales of this profile are not necessarily similar to those of the parent profile; they are derived from teachers' ratings of items differing somewhat from those that parents rate. However, even those items that are identical on the parent and teacher forms are not necessarily perceived to covary in the same way by parents and teachers. For example, even though teachers are asked to rate the same somatic complaints as parents, these did not covary to form a clearcut dimension as they did in the parent ratings. Conversely, even though parents are asked to rate items indicative of both inattention and overactivity, the parent ratings yielded a single dimension that we called Hyperactive, instead of the two dimensions called Inattentive and Nervous Overactive in the teacher ratings. Because parents and teachers do not necessarily perceive the same variations and covariations among behaviors, we cannot necessarily judge the accuracy of teachers' reports by comparison with parents' reports, nor vice versa.

Scott's teacher's ratings show important consistencies with his parents' ratings. Scott's total behavior problem score on the Teacher's Report was 93, which is well above the 90th percentile score of 49 for nonreferred six- to 11-year-old boys and in the range characteristic of many clinically referred boys. As shown by their ratings of a large pool of items, Scott's parents and teacher thus agree in perceiving considerably more problems than the parents and teachers of nonreferred boys.

More specifically, the teacher's ratings resemble those of Scott's parents in showing more deviance in the area of aggression than hyperactivity, despite the teacher's initial labeling of Scott as hyperactive. The teacher's ratings also show considerable deviance on the scales designated as Unpopular and Inattentive, which represent dimensions not found in parents' ratings. Teachers are typically better situated to judge behavioral variation in these characteristics than parents are.

The profiles obtained from the teacher and parent ratings show that Scott is viewed as having problems of aggression, overactivity, and withdrawal at both home and school. Problems of depression and delinquent behavior are seen mainly at home, whereas problems of unpopularity and inattentiveness are seen mainly at school. This is certainly a much more differentiated picture than would be gleaned from the initial referral complaint of hyperactivity, or from interviews with the parents or teacher; or probably from self-reports by Scott or direct observations, although we are also developing procedures to make taxometric use of self-reports and direct observations.

In formulating a treatment plan for Scott, we can explicitly target many more problems and competencies than if we had diagnosed him in terms of a particular nosological category; employed a unidimensional rating scale designed to provide a score for hyperactivity; made direct observations of his behavior where feasible; or arrived at either a psychodynamic or family dynamic formulation via psychological tests and interviews. By periodically readministering the taxometric instruments, we can also quantify change during and after the intervention, thereby detecting areas in which Scott may get worse as well as those in which he may improve.

If all this sounds prohibitively cumbersome and expensive, it is not. The primary taxometric data were obtained at no cost from Scott's parents and teacher and can be scored in a few minutes by a clerical worker or computer. Although this form of assessment does not replace all other necessary data, such as cognitive measures, medical examinations, and developmental histories, and it does not specifically tell us how to help Scott, it can provide us with a much clearer starting point for determining what interventions work best for whom and then monitoring the effects of these interventions with each child.

SUMMARY

So-called traditional approaches to assessment have focused largely on categorical diagnostic constructs. Behavioral assessment has focused on relatively molecular behaviors and environmental contingencies associated with them. Both approaches ultimately face the need to aggregate data across cases in order to form groupings of children or disorders from which to construct a generalizable knowledge base. This is the problem of *taxonomy*.

Although categorical conceptual paradigms have dominated taxonomic efforts, a *taxometric* paradigm might be advantageous at this stage in our understanding of child psychopathology, for several reasons:

1) To capitalize on quantitative methods for assessing and aggregating behaviors that vary quantitatively.

2) To provide a normative-developmental context in which to judge the behavior of individual children.
3) To derive typologies from quantitative variations in profile patterns.
4) To quantitatively assess each child's resemblance to such patterns.
5) To coordinate multiple perspectives that may each contribute valid data about children's functioning.

REFERENCES

ACHENBACH, T. M. (1978). The Child Behavior Profile: I. Boys aged 6-11. *Journal of Consulting and Clinical Psychology, 46,* 478-488.
ACHENBACH, T. M., & EDELBROCK, C. (1978). The classification of child psychopathology: A review and analysis of empirical efforts. *Psychological Bulletin, 85,* 1275-1301.
ACHENBACH, T. M., & EDELBROCK, C. (1981). Behavioral problems and competencies reported by parents of normal and disturbed children aged four through sixteen. *Monographs of the Society for Research in Child Development, 46* (Serial No. 188).
ACHENBACH, T. M., & EDELBROCK, C. (1983). *Manual for the Child Behavior Checklist and Revised Child Behavior Profile.* Burlington, VT: Department of Psychiatry, University of Vermont.
ACKERSON, L. (1942). *Children's behavior problems: Vol. 2. Relative importance and interrelations among traits.* Chicago: University of Chicago Press.
AMERICAN PSYCHIATRIC ASSOCIATION. (1980). *Diagnostic and statistical manual of mental disorders* (3rd edition). Washington, DC: American Psychiatric Association. (1st edition, 1952; 2nd edition, 1968).
BEITCHMAN, J. H., DIELMAN, T. E., LANDIS, J. R., BENSON, R. M., & KEMP, P. L. (1978). Reliability of the Group for the Advancement of Psychiatry diagnostic categories in child psychiatry. *Archives of General Psychiatry, 35,* 1461-1466.
EDELBROCK, C., & ACHENBACH, T. M. (1980). A typology of Child Behavior Profile patterns: Distribution and correlates in disturbed children aged 6 to 16. *Journal of Abnormal Child Psychology, 8,* 441-470.
EDELBROCK, C., & ACHENBCH, T. M. (1984). The Teacher Version of the Child Behavior Profile: I. Boys aged 6-11. *Journal of Consulting and Clinical Psychology, 52,* 207-217.
FREEMAN, M. (1971). A reliability study of psychiatric diagnosis in childhood and adolescence. *Journal of Child Psychology and Psychiatry, 12,* 43-54.
GROUP FOR THE ADVANCEMENT OF PSYCHIATRY. (1966). Psychopathological disorders in childhood: Theoretical considerations and a proposed classification (Vol. VI, *Report No. 62*). New York: Brunner/Mazel.
HEWITT, L. E., & JENKINS, R. L. (1946). *Fundamental patterns of maladjustment: The dynamics of their origin.* Springfield, IL: State of Illinois.
JENKINS, R. L., & GLICKMAN, S. (1946). Common syndromes in child psychiatry: I. Deviant Behavior Traits. II. The schizoid child. *American Journal of Orthopsychiatry, 16,* 244-261.
MASH, E. J., & TERDAL, L. G. (Eds.). (1981). *Behavioral assessment of childhood disorders.* New York: Guilford Press.
MATTISON, R., CANTWELL, D. P., RUSSELL, A. T., & WILL, L. (1979). A comparison of DSM-II and DSM-III in the diagnosis of childhood psychiatric disorders. *Archives of General Psychiatry, 36,* 1217-1222.
MEEHL, P. E., & GOLDEN, R. R. (1982). Taxometric methods. In P. C. Kendall & J. N. Butcher (Eds.), *Handbook of research methods in clinical psychology.* New York: Wiley.

MEZZICH, A. C., & MEZZICH, J. E. (1979). *Diagnostic reliability of childhood and adolescent behavior disorders.* Paper presented at the meeting of the American Psychological Association, New York, September 1979.

NAY, W. R. (1979). *Multimethod clinical assessment.* New York: Gardner Press.

PATTERSON, G. R. (1980). Mothers: The unacknowledged victims. *Monographs of the Society for Research in Child Development, 45* (Serial No. 186).

PATTERSON, G. R. (1981). Foreword. In E. J. Mash & L. G. Terdal (Eds.), *Behavioral assessment of childhood disorders.* New York: Guilford Press.

QUAY, H. C. (1979). Classification. In H. C. Quay & J. Werry (Eds.), *Psychopathological disorders of childhood* (2nd ed.). New York: Wiley.

RUTTER, M. & SHAFFER, D. (1980). DSM-III. A step forward or back in terms of the classification of child psychiatric disorders? *Journal of the American Academy of Child Psychiatry, 19,* 371-394.

RUTTER, M., SHAFFER, D., & SHEPHERD, M. (1975). *A multiaxial classification of child disorders: An evaluation of a proposal.* Geneva: World Health Organization.

SOKOL, R. R., & SNEATH, P. H. (1963). *Principles of numerical taxonomy.* San Francisco: Freeman.

WADE, T. C., BAKER, T. B., & HARTMANN, D. P. (1979). Behavior therapists' self-reported views and practices. *The Behavior Therapist, 2,* 3-6.

5
Parental Monitoring of Infant Development

DIANE BRICKER and
DAVID LITTMAN

INTRODUCTION

In the decade of the 80s, detection and intervention efforts have been broadened to include increasingly younger handicapped children (Bricker, 1981), infants medically at-risk (Friedman & Sigman, 1981), and infants environmentally at-risk (Ramey, MacPhee, & Yeates, 1983). The motivation for these trends appears to arise, in part, from a belief shared by many scientists, practitioners and parents that early intervention can be beneficial for handicapped infants and infants at-risk for developing serious problems. However, the value of early intervention has been questioned when offered as an isolated program

---

Support for this project is provided by a Grant from the National Institute for Handicapped Research, USOE, and the Center on Human Development, University of Oregon and by the cooperation of the administrative and NICU medical staff of Sacred Heart General Hospital, Eugene, Oregon and the administrative staff of the Center on Human Development. The authors wish to thank Ann Marie Jusczyk, Linda Mounts, Gail Cripe, and Linda Ficere for their efforts in collecting the data and the parents and infants who have participated in the project for providing it.

apart from the child's larger ecological context (Bronfenbrenner, 1975; Clarke & Clarke, 1977). In addition, others have questioned the value of early education directed to populations with genetic disorders such as Down's syndrome (Gibson & Fields, in press; Piper & Pless, 1980). On the other hand, advocates of early intervention may be overly confident about facilitative outcomes given the paucity of objective data to support their case. As a number of recent reviews note (see, for example, Bricker, Bailey, & Bruder, in press; Haskins, Finkelstein, & Stedman, 1978; Simeonsson, Cooper, & Scheiner, 1982; Stedman, 1977), the arguments put forth by critics and advocates neither accurately reflect the variety of outcomes found in the literature, nor do they constructively confront methodological problems inherent in intervention research (Baer, 1981).

Nonetheless, we are persuaded that the early intervention enterprise has gained sufficient support to maintain its place as an educational alternative for handicapped and at-risk infants and children, and that therefore, continuing efforts should be directed toward refining a range of intervention alternatives. A basic requisite for early intervention is a detection system that reliably discriminates infants and young children who are developing without problems from those who are not. Differentiation between populations who need assistance and those who do not is essential if limited and costly educational and therapeutic interventions are to be wisely deployed. Reliable screening and detection of organically handicapped infants is possible; however, in populations without overt physical or behavioral (e.g., motor impairments) symptoms, reliable detection remains a problem.

INFANT SCREENING AND DETECTION

Many serious developmental problems are not indicated by overt perinatal warning signs. Therefore, early detection and identification of infants with potentially serious problems are important issues for researchers and interventionists who believe benefits accrue from early intervention.

Although severe handicaps are usually recognized during the first weeks of life (Bricker & Dow, 1980; Hayden & Beck, 1982), efficient procedures for identifying infants with mild or moderate handicapping conditions or developmental problems have been more elusive (Haring, 1979; Meier, 1975; Scott & Masi, 1979). Many screening programs include the entire target population or a large subsample. In these programs the evaluation is extensive and is generally conducted by a multidisciplinary team. These approaches have high overscreening rates which make them costly and inefficient.

Research efforts addressing screening and detection have investigated prediction of future performance based on the infant's medical-biological status (Broman, 1979), behavioral functioning (Als, Lester, & Brazelton, 1979) or a combination of biological, behavioral and environmental variables (Sigman & Parmelee, 1979). These investigations are uniform in their findings that there is low predictive validity between infant behavior and biological characteristics during the first two years and later childhood functioning (Aylward & Kenny, 1979; Honzik, 1976). Interestingly, studies which have examined the dynamic interplay of biological, behavioral and environmental variables have resulted in better prediction of development (Ramey, Farran, & Campbell, 1979; Sameroff, 1981; Sigman & Parmelee, 1979). Unfortunately, moderately accurate prediction of mean outcomes for groups of at-risk infants does not necessarily provide accurate information about the status of individual babies (Parmelee, Kopp, & Sigman, 1976).

In addition to the problem of predicting the development of individual babies, Scott (1978) has pointed out that most proposed detection strategies would be prohibitively expensive. High per-child costs, particularly for infant populations of whom 70% may be normal, may be unacceptable to the general public.

The problem then is not only to identify infants with problems as early as possible, but to do so in a cost-effective manner. Two obvious points must be considered. First, it appears wise to concentrate screening and detection efforts on populations at increased risk for developing problems and second, to select techniques that can be implemented in an economical manner.

Ample research suggests that infants with prenatal and perinatal medical problems who require placement in a Newborn Intensive Care Unit (NICU) are at significantly greater risk for developing abnormally than infants with uneventful gestational and perinatal periods (Littman, 1979). However, not every infant who requires intensive perinatal medical care develops abnormally. Indeed, the majority of these infants develop without apparent problems. Scott and Masi (1979) estimate that only 30% of infants assigned to NICUs require some form of intervention by the first grade.* Because NICUs have a high percentage

---

* Even though, as Scott and Masi (1979) have pointed out, more handicapped children are actually in the group assigned to newborn nurseries, though the proportion is lower than in NICU.

of infants eventually requiring intervention, monitoring this population seems a fertile area for the development of a cost-effective method for the detection of infants who may require some form of intervention. Within the population of infants assigned to NICUs, the problem is to identify reliably the infants who will require intervention while avoiding the misclassification of the 70% who will develop without apparent problem.

THE USE OF PARENTS TO MONITOR THEIR INFANT'S DEVELOPMENT

Accurate, economical, long-term monitoring systems are needed for at-risk infants. Using parents to perform such monitoring with their infant provides an intriguing strategy that is worthy of exploration. The literature contains a few studies in which data were collected on agreement between parental and professional evaluations of the child (Donnelly, Doherty, Sheehan, & Whittemore, 1982; Gradel, Thompson, & Sheehan, 1981; Hunt & Paraskevopoulos, 1980). In general, these studies report good agreement between parental and professional evaluations with discrepancies tending to be in maternal overestimation of the child's performance, if one accepts the professional's judgment as the criterion.

Some of the most widely known work on infant screening has been done by Frankenburg and his colleagues. From the Denver Developmental Screening Test (Frankenburg & Dodds, 1967), the Prescreening Developmental Questionnaire (Frankenburg, Van Doorninck, Liddell, & Dick, 1976) was developed as a more efficient, and therefore more economical, procedure to prescreen large populations of infants. The Prescreening Developmental Questionnaire (PDQ) has 97 items (modified from DDST items) constructed to be answered by parents. These items are arranged in chronological order according to the age at which 90% of the children passed the item in the original DDST sample. Based on the child's age, parents answer 10 items from the PDQ. Children who are suspect are rescreened one to two weeks later. Using the PDQ this way requires one minute of professional time and costs three to five cents for the printed questionnaire. Frankenburg, Coons, and Ker (1982) report that the PDQ was more efficient in screening parent populations with high school educations, and the professionally administered DDST more efficient in screening less educated parent populations.

In 1979, Knobloch, Stevens, Malone, Ellison, and Risemberg reported a study on the validity of parental evaluation of their infants' development. A 36-item questionnaire with items derived from Gesell's Revised Developmental Screening Inventory (RDSI) representing the developmental period from 20 to 32 weeks was mailed to the parents of 526 28-week-old high-risk infants. The questionnaires were completed, returned, and scored to classify the babies as normal, abnormal, or questionable. At 40 weeks the infants were brought to the clinic for a professional developmental and neurological evaluation. When the questionnaire findings were compared with the full examination, Knobloch, Stevens, Malone, Ellison, and Risemberg (1979) reported that underscreening of abnormals was 2.6% (implying 97.4% accuracy), and underscreening of questionable (minor abnormalities) was 10% (implying accuracy of 90% in classifying normal babies correctly).

Knobloch et al. (1979) also provided an analysis of PDQ results reported by Frankenburg et al. (1976) which indicates that the PDQ detected 87% of the 30 abnormal children in Frankenburg's sample, 54% of the 106 questionable children, and 73% of the 1,005 normal children. These findings imply that the normal and questionable children were underscreened at a rate of 39%, while the normal children were overscreened by approximately 27% (and thus called abnormal or questionable). These screening rates, taken together, point up an important dilemma facing researchers and service delivery agencies. The PDQ identified 356 children as needing additional assessment; of these 356 children, only 23% were found to be abnormal. This outcome indicates that in order to identify one abnormal baby using the PDQ, it may be necessary to perform unnecessary professional evaluations on as many as three additional babies. In many settings, sufficient resources are not available to accommodate such overscreening rates. Even if resources are available, one must question their use in this manner.

Morse (1980) reported the results of a screening system designed to be administered to parents over the telephone. Morse compared her telephone screening system (the TIDS) with the DDSTR and PDQ, both of which were developed by Frankenburg. She reported that for the sample of 50 babies in the 10-month to 13.5-month age range, the TIDS completely agreed with the criterion diagnosis for abnormal babies based on a range of evaluation measures. The TIDS correctly classified all the abnormal children, 22% of the questionable children, and 74% of the normal children. The TIDS appears to have an overscreening rate similar to the rate for the PDQ. If this degree of overscreening is acceptable, the main advantages of the TIDS appear to lie in its ease of administration, its potential value as a screening instrument for use with illiterate populations, and the ease with which parental compliance with the screening system can be assured.

PURPOSE

Given the encouraging results reported by Frankenburg et al. (1982), Knobloch et al. (1979), and Morse (1980), the major purpose of our research was to determine the validity and cost of a longitudinal screening and monitoring system for a population of at-risk infants between 4 and 24 months of age. The monitoring system uses parents to complete questionnaires reflecting their infants' development at four, eight, 12, 16, 20, and 24 months. This approach draws heavily on the work of Knobloch et al. (1979) in that it employs parents to complete a questionnaire based on the RDSI. However, the screening system spans six test points and the congruence between parent and professional evaluations is, therefore, compared on six separate questionnaires rather than only at one point in time.

PROJECT OVERVIEW

Project Background

Early in 1980 a dialogue began between staff members of the Early Intervention Program at the University of Oregon's Center on Human Development, the medical staff of the Newborn Intensive Care Unit, Sacred Heart General Hospital in Eugene, Oregon,* the Crippled Children's Division of the University of Oregon Health Sciences Center,** and representatives of community agencies interested in following the development of infants discharged from the Newborn Intensive Care Unit (NICU) at Sacred Heart Hospital. Interest in such a project was strong among participants and this interest was realized when, in October, 1980, the National Institute for Handicapped Research funded the present project to examine cost-effective methods for monitoring, evaluating, and intervening with at-risk and handicapped infants.

The initial steps undertaken by the project staff were to develop cooperative liaisons between: 1) the NICU staff of Sacred Heart Gen-

---

* In particular, Drs. Jason Eliot and Carl Yaeger, the unit's neonatologists.
** In particular, Dr. Robert Nickel.

eral Hospital and the administrative personnel responsible for hospital operation; 2) the pediatric and medical community involved in delivering medical services to infants discharged from the NICU; 3) the Crippled Children's Division, the state agency primarily responsible for the evaluation of infants and children with developmental disabilities; and 4) other community health agencies that might be concerned with at-risk infants and their families.

Since cooperation with the NICU was essential to the success of the project, a series of meetings were held to design project procedures to be consonant with methods already used in the hospital's NICU. Since hospital approval was necessary before beginning the project, project staff provided appropriate information and attended meetings with hospital authorities to answer questions and describe the project. Support from the hospital's neonatologists as well as the developmental pediatrician from the Crippled Children's Division facilitated contacts with the general pediatric and medical community. Other community agencies were informed either through meetings or telephone contacts. Explanations of the project were provided, questions were answered and support was elicited from the various community organizations that might have contact with NICU infants and their parents.

Although the meetings and contacts were time-consuming, they were essential to the success of the project. Without support and assurance from the medical community and other agencies, parents would probably have been reluctant to participate. Cooperation from the NICU was essential to contacting families.

Initial Parental Contact

Two project staff members were authorized by Sacred Heart General Hospital to contact parents of NICU infants. Parents who were interested in learning about the project were approached by one of the two staff members shortly before the infant was discharged from the NICU. If the family chose to participate, a letter was sent to their physician informing him or her of the family's participation in the study. Subsequently, the physician was informed if the infant's development was found to be abnormal. Parents who decided not to participate were asked to complete a form indicating reasons for their decision. Families who decided to participate were told they would be contacted again, shortly before the infant reached four months of age.

Target Population

The target population came from the NICU of Sacred Heart General Hospital. This population was divided into four subgroups of infants and as Figure 1 shows, three of these subgroups of infants participated in the Infant Monitoring Project (IMP). Group O included infants who remained less than three days in the NICU and were excluded from the project. Many of the infants in Group O were assigned briefly to the NICU for transitory problems and all out-of-town infants who were transported to the hospital were initially placed in the NICU. The infants in Group O were not included since the purpose of the project was to track a group of infants who had a high probability of developing problems. The three-day criterion for exclusion was selected in consultation with the neonatologists and developmental pediatrician who served as medical consultants to this project.

Group 1 was composed of at-risk infants who remained in the NICU for at least three days. Group 2 infants were at extreme risk from medical complications. The criteria for this sample are presented in Table 1. After discharge from the NICU these infants were enrolled in the Newborn Follow-Up Clinic (NFC) administered by the Crippled Children's Division. Infants were evaluated in the NFC at four, eight, 12, 18, and 24 months. During the NFC visits the infants were assessed with the Revised Gesell and Amatruda Developmental and Neurological Examination (Knobloch, Stevens, & Malone, 1980) and the Movement Assessment of Infants (Chandler, Andrews, & Swanson, 1980).

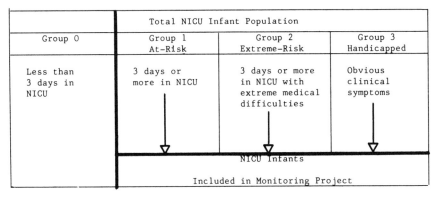

FIGURE 1. Subgroups of NICU infants

TABLE 1
Criteria for Assignment to Group 2
Extreme-Risk Infants Assigned to the Newborn Follow-up Clinic

Criteria	Description
1	CNS hemorrhage (includes sub-dural, intraventricular, and intracerebral)
2	Neonatal seizures (single prolonged, or multiple)
3	Neonatal asphyxia (Apgar less than four at five minutes)
4	Recurrent apnea requiring mechanical ventilation
5	SGA (less than 3rd percentile and less than 36 weeks gestation)
6	Birth weight less than 1,250 grams
7	CNS infection (meningitis and encephalitis)
8	Intrauterine infection (CMV, toxoplasmosis, etc.)
9	RDS with mechanical ventilation and "neurologic abnormality"*
10	Hyperbilirubinemia and "neurologic abnormality"*
11	Hypoglycemia and "neurologic abnormality"*
12	Birth trauma and "neurologic abnormality"*
13	CNS malformation (includes hydrocephalus, microcephaly, encephalocele, etc.)

*"Neurologic abnormality" refers to the primary physician's clinical impression that the infant has a global neurologic dysfunction near time of discharge, and includes: continued lethargy with hypokinesis and feeding difficulties due to a poor suck (apathy syndrome); hypotonia; hypertonia, especially with opisthotonic posturing; and three or more consistent asymmetries in exam (hemi syndrome), especially when combined with other signs such as hypotonia, hypertonia, or hyperexcitability.

Group 3 consisted of infants with identifiable handicaps. Although these infants had known problems, a small number were included as an additional check on the validity of the questionnaire system.

Figure 2 provides an illustration of the infants' movement from the NICU to their appropriate group assignment for participation in the project. Those infants identified as disabled were referred for intervention services.

Parents of local infants were asked to bring the infant to the Center at four-month intervals that coincided with their completion of the mailed questionnaire. During the visit to the Center the infant was given a full-scale Gesell by a trained examiner. This group of infants comprised the largest subject pool for the investigation. Parents of the remaining infants (generally nonlocal) were asked to bring their infant to the Center for testing only if the infant's reported performance on the questionnaire was abnormal or questionable on two consecutive questionnaires.

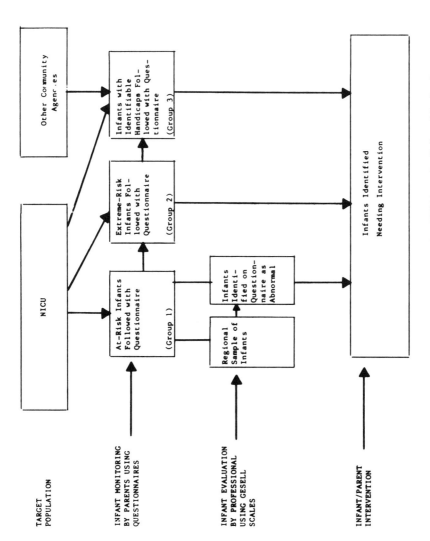

FIGURE 2. Schematic of infants' movement from the NICU to the Infant Monitoring Project

The Parent Monitoring Questionnaires

Pilot studies (Gruhn, 1981; Nelson, 1981; Sims, 1982) with the four, eight, 20, and 24-month questionnaires suggested several format changes. The finalized monitoring system includes six questionnaires to be completed by parents when the infant is four, eight, 12, 16, 20, and 24 months of age (corrected age was used for premature infants).

The cover sheet for each questionnaire asks parents for identifying information (e.g., name, date, person completing the questionnaire, etc.) and provides instructions for completion. Each of the six questionnaires is identical in format and includes five assessment categories: 1) communication, 2) gross motor, 3) fine motor, 4) adaptive, and 5) personal-social. The final page asks five general questions (e.g., Has your child had trouble eating or sleeping?). The content of the questionnaires was derived largely from the Revised Gesell Scales (Knobloch et al., 1980) and the Revised Parent Developmental Questionnaire (Knobloch et al., 1980), although other sources were used to construct the 16, 20, and 24-month questionnaire.

Each questionnaire has a total of 35 questions divided equally among the five areas. Each of the five assessment categories contains seven items; six of these items cover the developmental quotient range of 75 to 100. The rationale for choosing this range is that infants performing at or above the norm (e.g., 100) are probably developing without problems. The decision to limit the D.Q. range from 75 to 100 also shortened the questionnaires, enhancing their attractiveness as a screening instrument. Each of the five domains contains one item with a D.Q. of 150. This item was included to provide some information about parents' tendencies to overestimate their infants' development—a reported parental phenomenon (Hunt & Paraskevopoulos, 1980; Gradel et al., 1981).

To avoid cumbersome language of "his/her" on the same questionnaire, female and male forms of the questionnaire were developed. Illustrations of the target action (e.g., the infant can sit independently) were included to clarify some items. The questionnaires are in a mailback format that is folded, addressed and stamped.

For each of the items on each of the five scales, parents could check "yes" indicating they believed the baby performs the behavior, "sometimes" indicating occasional performance of the response, or "not yet" indicating they believed the baby does not perform the behavior. Currently, the PMQ is scored as follows: Each category is assigned a cutoff point for abnormal. Scoring less than or equal to this cut-off classifies the baby's performance on that scale as abnormal. Current abnormal cut-offs for the 4-month questionnaire are 2.5 points for the communication scale, 4.5 points for the gross motor scale, 2.5 points for the fine motor scale, 3.5 points for the adaptive scale, and 3 points for the personal-social scale. For the 8-month questionnaire, current cut-offs are 3 points, 4 points, 4 points, 2.5 points, and 2.5 points for the same scales given as above. With the individual scales classified as normal, abnormal or questionable an overall classification was assigned based on the number of scales on which a child's performance was abnormal. If the child performed abnormally on one or more scales, then an overall classification of abnormal was assigned. Questionable scores on more than three scales also led to an overall classification of abnormal. Three questionable scores led to a questionable overall rating, and a normal overall classification was assigned if the child received no more than two questionable ratings and no abnormal ratings. If the infant received a single abnormal overall classification or two consecutive questionable classifications, then the parents were asked to bring the infant to the Center for further evaluation.

It is possible that parents' accuracy in completing the questionnaire is dependent on certain parental characteristics. We suspect, as have others (for example, Frankenburg, 1981), that not all parents will be able to monitor their at-risk infants successfully with a questionnaire. To determine which parental characteristics or social and economic factors are associated with the ability to use the questionnaire, each family was asked to complete a demographic form which requested specific, objective information. Any response that required speculation or subjectivity on the part of the parent was eliminated from the demographic form. These data provide a set of objective variables which may be useful in determining ability to use the questionnaire successfully.

PROCEDURES

After an infant had been in the NICU at least three days and his or her condition was stable, the parents were approached about the Infant Monitoring Project (IMP). Parents who indicated an interest in the study were contacted by the project's Infant Development Specialist (IDS). The IDS made arrangements to visit the parents at the hospital before the infant was discharged. During this visit the project was described, written consent obtained, and the demographic form completed. Parents for whom a hospital meeting was not possible were contacted by phone. A notification letter was sent to the infant's pediatrician or physician stating that the family was participating in the study.

If parents chose not to participate, attempts were made to collect data on reasons for non-participation. Attempts were made to gather these data from parents who requested further information initially and then chose not to participate. However, many of these parents did not return the questionnaire seeking their reasons for non-participation. Such data were not collected on infants whose parents were not contacted on advice of the NICU medical consultants (due to severe medical complications), the NICU social worker (acute family problems or adoption cases), or parents who initially refused to participate.

Four months after the infant's birth (age corrected for prematurity if necessary) and at four-month intervals thereafter to 24 months, the parents received the infant monitoring questionnaires by mail. For infants who lived outside the local area, parents were sent the appropriate questionnaire seven working days before the infant became four, eight, 12, 16, 20, or 24 months of age. The IDS telephoned the parents five days after the questionnaire was sent to explain how to complete it. If the questionnaire was not returned by a specific time, parents were telephoned and offered assistance in completing the questionnaire with the option of completing it over the telephone.

Initially, infants in the local area received home visits within 14 days of becoming four months corrected age. Parents were contacted by telephone 14 working days before the infant was four months old. Parents were informed of the reason for the home visit (to give instructions for completing the questionnaire, and to complete other assessment measures if they were willing to do so). The home visit took about an hour and was arranged at the parents' convenience when the baby was likely to be awake. Parents received a reminder phone call the day before the scheduled home visit. The primary reason for including home visits was to maintain family participation. However, an analysis of the attrition data 20 months after the project began indicated little difference in attrition rates between families receiving home visits and those not receiving visits. Because the home visits were expensive to maintain and appeared not to be affecting the rate of participation, they were discontinued.

Once a questionnaire was returned by the parents, it was scored to determine a classification for the infant. The results of the scoring for an infant yielded one of three ratings: normal, questionable, or abnormal. For infants falling into the normal category on the PMQ and who either received no Gesell or were rated as normal on the Gesell, parents were sent letters indicating that the infant was developing as expected. The same procedure was followed for infants receiving a questionable rating unless the infant received two consecutive questionable ratings. If this occurred or the infant received an abnormal rating, the parents were invited to bring the infant to the Center for further testing. This procedure was followed with all infants who received a rating that indicated further evaluation was in order.

The Center evaluation was scheduled whenever possible within a period of two weeks of the receipt of the parents' questionnaire in order to optimize the comparison between the standardized measure used by the professional and the questionnaire completed by the parent. The parents brought the infant to the Center, were greeted by the IDS and escorted to a small, but pleasant testing room. Once the infant and parents were relatively comfortable, the assessment using the Gesell was begun. The IDS followed the procedure specified in the Gesell manual (Knobloch et al., 1980). The infant's response to each item was recorded. Following the completion of the test, the parents were given a general idea of how their child performed. Within the next day the Gesell protocol was scored and if the infant's performance was in the abnormal range, the family's private physician was informed. If the physician desired, the IDS also contacted the parents. After being alerted that the infant was found to be in the abnormal range, the general procedure was that either the parent or the physician, or both, contacted the Crippled Children's Division to request a full-scale evaluation that was conducted by a multidisciplinary team.

RESULTS

Sample

Table 2 presents education, income, and occupational data on the total project sample. The distribution of educational levels for main wage earners and mothers is contained in Table 2. These data indicate the sample has generally either high school or college experience. Table 2 also shows considerable uniformity in the distribution of income for the population. The occupational composition, as shown in Table 2, ranged from unskilled workers to administrative personnel. These demographic statistics suggest our sample was similar, in these respects,

TABLE 2

Percent Distribution of Education, Annual Income and Occupation of Families Participating in the Infant Monitoring Project

Overall Category	*Sub-Categories of Education*					
	Jr. High School	Some High School	High School	Some College	College	Graduate School
N = 271						
Education of Main Wage Earner	.01	.10	.32	.31	.21	.04
Mother's Education	.04	.13	.35	.27	.18	.03

	Sub-Categories of Annual Income					
	<$5,000	$5-$10,000	$10-$15,000	$15-$20,000	$20-$25,000	>$25,000
Annual Family Income	.10	.20	.15	.25	.14	.16

	Sub-Categories of Occupation						
	Executive	Business Manager	Administrative Personnel	Clerical	Skilled Manual	Machine Operator	Unskilled
Occupation of Main Wage Earner	.02	.07	.23	.21	.12	.19	.15

to that of Frankenburg et al. (1976). Ninety-five percent of the mothers were between 18 and 39 years of age at the time of the infant's birth. Data on marital status shows that 7% were single, 89% had partners and 4% were involved in extended families but without a partner. Fifty-nine percent of the infant sample were male while 41% were female. Approximately 64% of the sample were premature and 4% were postmature.

The disposition of all eligible infants who spent time in the NICU during the project is of interest. Of the approximately 450 families (multiple births occurred), the project contacted 425. Of these, 329 agreed to participate. Of those who agreed to participate, 44 dropped out of the study. This left a sample of 285 infants and their families. Reasons families gave for their discontinuation in the project were classified as justified or unjustified. A classification of justified was assigned if the infant died, the family moved out of state, or a family crisis occurred such as the mother becoming hospitalized. Unjustified reasons included losing interest, no longer wanting to participate, not having adequate time, not returning forms or telephone calls, and so forth. Using this classification system, 19 of the 44 families' reasons were found to be unjustified. This means that of the original group who agreed to participate, only 5% left the project for reasons that did not seem justified.

Screening

The effectiveness of the PMQ as a screening instrument is presented first for the combined regional and NFC samples and then for three subsamples to clarify the nature of the screening results. This project is still underway and currently an adequate sample is available for only the four- and eight-month time periods; therefore, results on the 12, 16, 20, and 24 month periods are not reported. In addition, the parental evaluation of the infant's performance on the items with 150 D.Q. were excluded from the analyses because several infants were observed to perform these behaviors during the Gesell testing.

Total Combined Regional and NFC Sample

Screening results for the combined regional and NFC sample at four and eight months are presented in Table 3. Results of Gesell examinations were used to classify infants as follows: If the infant received a score of less than 75 in a single category, he or she was classified as

TABLE 3

Percent Agreement and Disagreement of the PMQ Classification with Gesell Classification at Four- and Eight-Month Test for Combined NFC and Regional Sample

	Gesell Classifications			
	Abnormal or Questionable		Normal	
	Agree	Disagree	Agree	Disagree
4 months (N = 100)				
Percent	.55	.45	.82	.18
Number of Infants	16/29	13/29	58/71	13/71
8 months (N = 68)				
Percent	.86	.14	.85	.15
Number of Infants	6/7	1/7	52/61	9/61

abnormal; if a single scale led to a score between 75 and 84, then the infant was classified as questionable; otherwise the infant was classified as normal. Parent Monitoring Questionnaire classifications were made as described above.

The primary question of interest was whether the PMQ could detect questionable or abnormal children using the Gesell as the criterion measure. Therefore, the abnormal and questionable categories were collapsed and screening rates were calculated for the normal and questionable/abnormal groups. At four months, when using the Gesell as the criterion measure, the questionnaire seems to have an underscreening rate of 45% while having an overscreening rate of 18%. At eight months, overscreening drops to 15%, while underscreening was reduced to 14%.

Detection of six of the seven abnormal or questionable infants by the PMQ at eight months was significant beyond the 5% level by binomial test. Of importance is the shift in the number of infants classified by the Gesell as abnormal at four months but normal at the eight-month test period. If these infants maintain their normal status at future test periods, it appears that the Gesell may have overscreened these particular infants. That is, the Gesell may have been less accurate than parents in prognostic evaluation of the infants at least from four to eight months. This possibility is supported because, of the 29 abnormal or questionable babies in the four-month sample, 12 infants were classified as abnormal because of poor performance on a single scale (e.g., the Gross Motor Scale, the adaptive scale). Of the 12 infants classified at four months as abnormal on a single scale according to the Gesell, eight were given abnormal scores on the Gross Motor Scale. Of these eight babies, seven were in the NFC and one was in the regional subsample. At eight months, only one infant in this group, an NFC baby, still was given an abnormal score on the Gross Motor Scale, three were classified as normal, and three were classified as questionable. One baby's data were missing at eight months. Of the seven babies without missing data, five received some form of intervention. This was principally physical therapy.

Newborn Follow-Up Clinic Subsample

These infants, who were deemed by the developmental pediatrician to be at extreme risk based on the criteria contained in Table 1, were placed in a follow-up program immediately upon discharge from the NICU. Table 4 presents the screening results for this subsample at

TABLE 4

Percent Agreement and Disagreement of the PMQ Classification with the Gesell Classification at Four and Eight Months for the Newborn Follow-Up Sample and Regional Sample

| | Gesell Classifications Newborn Follow-Up Sample | | | |
| | Abnormal or Questionable | | Normal | |
	Agree	Disagree	Agree	Disagree
4 months (N = 46)				
Percent	.48	.52	.76	.24
Number of Infants	10/21	11/21	19/25	6/25
8 months (N = 30)				
Percent	.80	.20	.80	.20
Number of Infants	4/5	1/5	20/25	5/25
Regional Sample				
4 months (N = 54)				
Percent	.75	.25	.85	.15
Number of Infants	6/8	2/8	39/46	7/46
8 months (N = 38)				
Percent	1.0	—	.89	.11
Number of Infants	2/2	—	32/36	4/36

four and eight months. The pattern of underscreening at four months and accurate screening at eight months seen in the full sample is replicated in this group. In fact, of the seven abnormal or questionable infants in the total sample at eight months, five of them were in the NFC population. This means that of the two abnormal or questionable infants *not* in the NFC at eight months, both were detected by the PMQ. Of the five infants remaining in the NFC, four were detected. Overscreening rates are marginally higher in the NFC subsample compared to the total sample; this is not surprising given the small size and extreme risk of the sample.

Regional Subsample

The regional subsample was composed of the babies in the NICU population whose families lived within approximately 20 miles of the Eugene metropolitan area and excluded the NFC infants and infants who lived beyond the metropolitan area. The screening results for the regional subsample, presented in Table 4, show that the PMQ detected 75% of those considered to be abnormal or questionable at four months. This figure is significant at the 5% level by binomial test. Overscreening was held to 15%. The screening picture at eight months is encouraging in that all abnormal babies were detected by the PMQ and the overscreening rate was 11%.

Screened Subsample

The screened subsample included all infants who were not part of either the NFC or the regional subsample, but whose parents were completing the PMQ. In general these were families who lived beyond the metropolitan area. When a PMQ from this sample was received that indicated the infant was abnormal or had two questionable ratings, the parent was asked to bring the infant to the Center for further testing. This subsample may parallel most closely the group of infants without obvious problems who confront a service delivery system using an infant screening system. At four months there were four babies who were identified by the PMQ as questionable or abnormal. All four were classified as abnormal by the Gesell. At eight months one additional infant was detected by the PMQ. This infant was also classified as abnormal by the Gesell.

Discussion

The main question of interest is, of course, whether infant screening as implemented by the Parent Monitoring Questionnaire system is effective. To answer this question it is necessary to define carefully what is meant by "effective."

If by effective we mean the PMQ classification agrees with the Gesell on 95% of the babies at all test points, then the answer based on the four- and eight-month data is "no." The underscreening rates at four months ranged from 45% for the total sample to 52% for the Newborn Follow-Up Subsample. This suggests that the parental responses to the PMQ cannot be scored so that the classifications of nearly all infants by the PMQ and the Gesell will be the same. The present findings indicate that to avoid any underscreening at four months, it would be necessary to overscreen at a high rate, similar to the rate required by Frankenburg's PDQ to identify most abnormal infants (recall that the PDQ overscreened three infants in order to catch one abnormal infant).

If by effective we mean that the PMQ is able to identify most infants who appear to be at-risk by some critical test age, say eight months, then the answer appears to be "yes." The underscreening rate in the total sample was very low and, just as important, the overscreening rate was quite modest. Of interest is the apparent discrepancy between classification by parents and professionals.

Possible explanations for this discrepancy are numerous. First, the responses that caused the professional examiner to classify the infant as abnormal or questionable at four months may be responses that are present rather than responses that are absent; for example, reflexes that should be absent but are not, or excessive muscle tone that parents may not be able to discriminate. By eight months the reflexes may have been eliminated and the excess muscle tone become more normal resulting in the infant's reclassification by the professional examiner. A second possibility is that the professional examiner may be better at detecting more subtle responses or important response gradations than parents. Detection of these subtle variations may result in a difference in classification. Third, the parent has the opportunity to evaluate the infant using a vastly larger sample of behavior. In comparison, the professional examiner observed the infant for a relatively short time and was forced to make judgments on that small sample of behavior. There may be other reasons that would illuminate the discrepancy in classification between parents and professionals. Isolation of the appropriate explanation or explanations becomes important given the proportion of infants whose shift in Gesell classification at eight months more accurately reflected the parent's classification of these infants at four months. We intend to identify this group of infants and follow their developmental progress at 12, 16, 20, and 24 months.

The outcome from this project at four and eight months poses an important question; namely, how do we evaluate the effectiveness of a screening system designed to detect infants at-risk for developmental problems? To answer this question meaningfully, the goals of the screening system must be made explicit. Is the goal to monitor the development of a select group of infants? If so, the questionnaire system seems well suited to this task since parents appear to enjoy the contact with the monitoring project (cf. low attrition rates). In addition to the comfort parents feel with the system, completing the questionnaires may be a form of intervention. The activity of using the questionnaire may alert the parents to aspects of the infant's behavior that might otherwise be overlooked.

If the goal of the screening system is to provide a method for detecting infants *who will then be directed to intervention programs,* then the problems of underscreening and overscreening must be confronted. As a first step, the organization implementing the screening system must evaluate its resources. If the resources of the screening organization are extensive, which means that it can provide intervention for every baby who requires help, then the appropriate strategy would be to overscreen in order to detect and provide help for every baby needing it. Unfortunately, it seems unlikely that many organizations will be in such an enviable position in the near future.

If the resources of the service system are limited, a large number of overscreening errors may be unacceptable. In these circumstances the most appropriate strategy is to underscreen, running the risk of missing babies needing help, but being sure that the babies being detected are in need of intervention.

Results from this investigation, as well as data from other studies, make clear the dilemma inherent in screening programs for at-risk infants. For a variety of reasons, no system is likely to be found that always correctly discriminates among categories of infants. First, criterion measures may be in error. That is, the selected criterion measure may misclassify some infants. Second, development is dynamic and thus the infant's classification can be legitimately different at different points in time. Third, the screening instrument's accuracy may be differentially affected by the user. Some users will be able to employ reliably the screening measure while others may not. Do these problems render screening systems invalid? Clearly not, as the outcomes of this investigation indicate that considerable congruence between parental and professional evaluation is possible; however, disagreements also exist.

Knowing that the instrument underscreens abnormal and questionable infants and overscreens normal infants at four months, yet seems to be quite accurate at eight months, should lead to placing more weight on the results of the eight-month questionnaire. If resources are severely limited, then perhaps it would be reasonable for an agency to pick only the most clearly abnormal infants at early test points (employing an analogue of the triage system used to deliver emergency medical care when all victims cannot be served) and delaying decisions for most infants until they are eight or 12 months old.

Given a screening-detection system that is generally valid (e.g., adequate congruence with the criterion measure exists), the trick then is to adjust the scoring of the screening system to arrive at acceptable rates of underscreening and overscreening to meet the resources of the particular agency or program implementing the system.

In addition to determining acceptable underscreening and overscreening rates, most agencies and programs interested in monitoring at-risk populations are concerned with a cost/benefit analysis of the system. Cost data collected for the PMQ indicate the system is relatively inexpensive to maintain. The cost per infant per questionnaire is approximately $2.50. The cost is composed of two distinct components. First, the cost of materials (the printed questionnaire and postage) amounted to approximately 50 cents. The additional cost was incurred by administrative activities required to maintain and update subject lists, mail out and score questionnaires, and inform parents and physicians of the results. This total includes all costs encountered in maintaining the tracking system but does not include the costs of further evaluation of the infant. If resources are not limited and effective intervention can be provided to many infants, then the cost/benefit analysis should set a relatively lax criterion for providing further evaluation and services for a baby. Whether resources are limited or not, the screening will be most effective when there is congruence between the screening system, program goals, resources, and the service plan of an agency.

Behavioral scientists as well as practitioners must face the message being voiced by the vocal majority of citizens of this country—social and educational programs for the poor and disabled will no longer receive the fiscal support they enjoyed during the 60s and 70s. Facing this reality is unpleasant but to do otherwise seems unconscionable. At stake is the development of many of our children. This demands wise and judicious use of limited resources for individuals in need of assistance. It is therefore necessary to develop service models to provide high quality intervention in a cost-effective manner. A critical link is a reliable and cost-effective system to identify infants in need of assistance. The initial data collected on the parent-completed questionnaires described in this chapter suggest this tool may have the potential to offer such a link.

REFERENCES

ALS, H., LESTER, B., & BRAZELTON, T. (1979). Dynamics of the behavior organization of the premature infant: A theoretical perspective. In T. Field, A. Sostek, S. Goldberg, & H. Shuman (Eds.), *Infants born at risk*. Jamaica, NY: Spectrum Publications.

AYLWARD, G., & KENNY, T. (1979). Developmental follow-up: Inherent problems and a conceptual model. *Journal of Pediatric Psychology, 4*, 331-343.

BAER, D. (1981). The nature of intervention research. In R. Schiefelbusch & D. Bricker (Eds.), *Early language: Acquisition and intervention*. Baltimore, MD: University Park Press.

BRICKER, D. (1981). Preschool program, Center on Human Development, University of Oregon. Final report to the Division of Innovation and Development, U.S. Office of Education, Washington, D.C.

BRICKER, D., BAILEY, E., & BRUDER, M. (in press). The efficacy of early intervention and the handicapped infant: A wise or wasted resource? *Advances in Developmental and Behavioral Pediatrics* (Vol. 5). Greenwich, CT: JAI Press.

BRICKER, D., & DOW, M. (1980). Early intervention with the young severely handicapped child. *Journal of the Association for the Severely Handicapped, 5*, 130-142.

BROMAN, S. (1979). Prenatal anoxia and cognitive development. In T. Field, A. Sostek, S. Goldberg, & H. Shuman (Eds.), *Infants born at risk*. Jamaica, NY: Spectrum Publications.

BRONFENBRENNER, U. (1975). Is early intervention effective? In B. Friedlander, G. Sterritt, & G. Kirk (Eds.), *Exceptional infant: Assessment and intervention* (Vol. 3). New York: Brunner/Mazel.

CHANDLER, L., ANDREWS, M., & SWANSON, M. (1980). *Movement assessment of infants: A manual*. University of Washington, Seattle, Washington.

CLARKE, A., & CLARKE, A. (1977). Prospects for prevention and amelioration of mental retardation: A guest editorial. *American Journal of Mental Deficiency, 81*, 523-533.

DONNELLY, B., DOHERTY, J., SHEEHAN, R., & WHITTEMORE, C. (1982, December). *A comparison of maternal, paternal, and diagnostic evaluations of typical and atypical infants*. Paper presented at HCEEP/DEC Conference, Washington, D.C.

FRANKENBURG, W. (1981). Early screening for developmental delays and potential school problems. In C. Brown (Ed.), *Infants at risk*. Johnson & Johnson Baby Products Company.

FRANKENBURG, W., COONS, C., & KER, C. (1982). Screening infants and preschoolers to identify school learning problems. In E. Edgar, N. Haring, J. Jenkins, & C. Pious (Eds.), *Mentally handicapped children*. Baltimore, MD: University Park Press.

FRANKENBURG, W., & DODDS, J. (1967). The Denver Developmental Screening Test. *Journal of Pediatrics, 71,* 181-191.

FRANKENBURG, W., VAN DOORNINCK, W., LIDDELL, T., & DICK, N. (1976). The Denver prescreening developmental questionnaire (PDQ). *Pediatrics, 57,* 744-753.

FRIEDMAN, S., & SIGMAN, M. (Eds.). (1981). *Preterm birth and psychological development.* New York: Academic Press.

GIBSON, D., & FIELDS, D. (in press). Early stimulation programs for Down's syndrome: An effectiveness inventory. *Advances in Developmental and Behavioral Pediatrics* (Vol. 5). Greenwich, CT: JAI Press.

GRADEL, K., THOMPSON, M., & SHEEHAN, R. (1981). Parental and professional agreement in early childhood assessment. *Topics in Early Childhood Special Education, 1,* 31-40.

GRUHN, S. (1981). *A field test of the infant monitoring questionnaire for eight-month-old infants.* Unpublished masters thesis, University of Oregon.

HARING, N. (1979). Foreword. In B. Darby & M. May (Eds.), *Infant assessment: Issues and application.* Seattle: WESTAR.

HASKINS, R., FINKELSTEIN, N., & STEDMAN, D. (1978). Infant stimulation programs and their effects. *Pediatric Annals, 7,* 123-144.

HAYDEN, A., & BECK, G. (1982). The epidemiology of high-risk and handicapped infants. In C. Ramey & P. Trohanis (Eds.), *Finding and educating high-risk and handicapped infants.* Baltimore, MD: University Park Press.

HONZIK, M. (1976). Value and limitations of infant tests: An overview. In M. Lewis (Ed.), *Origins of intelligence.* New York: Plenum Press.

HUNT, J., & PARASKEVOPOULOS, J. (1980). Children's psychological development as a function of the accuracy of their mothers' knowledge of their abilities. *The Journal of Genetic Psychology, 136,* 285-298.

KNOBLOCH, H., STEVENS, F., & MALONE, A. (1980). *Manual of developmental diagnosis: The administration and interpretation of the revised Gesell and Amatruda developmental and neurologic examination.* Hagerstown: Harper & Row.

KNOBLOCH, H., STEVENS, F., MALONE, A., ELLISON, P., & RISEMBERG, H. (1979). The validity of parental reporting of infant development. *Pediatrics, 63,* 873-878.

LITTMAN, B. (1979). The relationship of medical events to infant development. In T. Field, A. Sostek, S. Goldberg, & H. Shuman (Eds.), *Infants born at risk.* Jamaica, NY: Spectrum Publications.

MEIER, J. (1975). Screening, assessment, and intervention for young children at developmental risk. In B. Friedlander, G. Sterritt, & G. Kirk (Eds.), *Exceptional infant: Assessment and intervention* (Vol. 3). New York: Brunner/Mazel.

MORSE, K. (1980). Telephone interview for developmental screening: A validity study. *Physical and Occupational Therapy in Pediatrics, 1,* 11-30.

NELSON, D. (1981). *Developmental assessment of infants by their primary caregivers: A pilot study of reliability and attitudes.* Unpublished masters thesis, University of Oregon.

PARMELEE, A., KOPP, C., & SIGMAN, M. (1976). Selection of developmental assessment techniques for infants at risk. *Merrill-Palmer Quarterly, 22,* 177-199.

PIPER, M., & PLESS, I. (1980). Early intervention for infants with Down's syndrome: A controlled trial. *Pediatrics, 65,* 463-468.

RAMEY, C., FARRAN, D., & CAMPBELL, F. (1979). Early intervention: From research to practice. In B. Darby & M. May (Eds.), *Infant assessment: Issues and applications.* Seattle: WESTAR.

RAMEY, C., MACPHEE, D., & YEATES, K. (1983). Preventing developmental retardation: A general systems model. In L. Bond & J. Joffe (Eds.), *Facilitating infant and early childhood development.* Hanover, NH: University Press of New England.

SAMEROFF, A. (1981). Longitudinal studies of preterm infants: A review of chapters 17-20. In S. Friedman & M. Sigman (Eds.), *Preterm birth and psychological development.* New York: Academic Press.

SCOTT, K. (1978). The rationale and methodological considerations underlying early cognitive and behavioral assessment. In F. Minifie & L. Lloyd (Eds.), *Communicative and cognitive abilities—early behavioral assessment.* Baltimore: University Park Press.

SCOTT, K., & MASI, W. (1979). The outcome from the utility of registers of risk. In T. Field, A. Sostek, S. Goldberg, & H. Shuman (Eds.), *Infants born at risk.* Jamaica, NY: Spectrum Publications.

SIGMAN, M., & PARMELEE, A. (1979). Longitudinal evaluation of the preterm infant. In T. Field, A. Sostek, S. Goldberg, & H. Shuman (Eds.), *Infants born at risk.* Jamaica, NY: Spectrum Publications.

SIMEONSSON, R., COOPER, D., & SCHEINER, A. (1982). A review and analysis of the effectiveness of early intervention programs. *Pediatrics, 69,* 635-641.

SIMS, C. (1982). *A pilot study of two parent administered developmental questionnaires.* Unpublished masters thesis, University of Oregon, 1982.

STEDMAN, D. (1977). Important considerations in the review and evaluation of educational intervention programs. In P. Mittler (Ed.), *Research to practice in mental retardation: Care and intervention* (Vol. 1). Baltimore, MD: University Park Press.

6
The Integration of Exceptional Children Within Preschool Environments: A Decision-Making Model

GERARD M. KYSELA, SALLY BARROS,
NANCY C. GRIGG, and MARILYN KANEE

The integration of young exceptional children (handicapped physically, intellectually, or socio-emotionally) into "regular" preschool programs with their normally developing peers has been an increasingly popular educational alternative in the last decade. The rationale for this significant shift in the provision of educational services is based on a complex set of philosophical and ideological issues, as well as numerous assumptions concerning the positive effects of these programs, not only for the handicapped child and his or her parents, but for the nonhandicapped peers and their parents, the school personnel

This research was supported by the Faculty of Education, The University of Alberta and Alberta Social Services and Community Health, through the McCalla Research Professorship to the first author and research grants for projects in this field from Alberta Social Services.

and, eventually, the community at large. However, a review of the literature reveals that, to a large extent, no empirical evidence has been produced in support of these assumptions.

It should also be noted that there is little consensus in the research literature concerning the operational definition of integration. It is clear, however, that integration is a very complex process, involving far more than the mere physical placement of the handicapped child in the classroom. For the purpose of this chapter, the term integration is defined as the placement of exceptional children within typical or "normal" school environments for all or some portion of their educational day as a means of providing an appropriate degree of social, instructional, and temporal contact with the normally developing age mates (Kaufman, Gottlieb, Agard, & Kukic, 1975). A range of options for the individualized education of exceptional students should be available from which appropriate experiences are selected and provided relative to the students' needs and the resources available from the program/school. The primary goal of integration or mainstreaming would be the provision of an appropriate educational experience for the exceptional child, not the total integration of all exceptional students into the learning environment.

For the purposes of this discussion, the exceptional individual is defined as a child who essentially perceives, learns, develops and remembers through similar processes as the normal child but does so at a different rate or via different routes than the normal or typical person (Telford & Sawrey, 1981). Obvious exceptions to this notion of exceptionality would be in domains in which biological/structural deficiencies or disabilities are evident. This conceptualization of exceptionality emphasizes the quantitative differences between exceptional children and normal children in such areas as physical growth, problem solving skills, attitudes, or emotional behavior patterns.

The process of integration then will require careful planning and program preparation to satisfy the unique needs of each individual exceptional child (Safford & Rosen, 1981). In order to maintain a consistent and equitable approach to the system's preparation for the integration of exceptional children, an organized and thorough decision-making plan seems essential, particularly to ensure attention to and planning for each facet of the integration process (Meisels, 1977). Following a brief statement of rationale, a decision-making model will be presented which attempts to meet the need to plan and implement effective integration.

RATIONALE FOR INTEGRATION

Over the past several decades, beginning with Dunn's (1968) classic review of segregated/integrated school placements, there has been a worldwide trend away from segregated school placements for exceptional children (Ackerman & Moore, 1976; Wilton & Densem, 1977). In fact, in a recent article examining the efficacy of special education compared to regular classes, Carlberg and Kovale (1980) reaffirmed, using a meta-analysis technique encompassing several studies, that integrated class placement was as successful for exceptional children with low I.Q. as segregated class placement. Despite this, Carlberg and Kovale (1980) and others (Blacher-Dixon, Leonard, & Turnbull, 1981; Meisels, 1977) feel that the policy of integration is in advance of extant analyses and support from empirical research.

Five major points arise when considering the logic for supporting integration of exceptional children within preschool programs:

1) The goals of early integration of exceptional children include stigma reduction/removal associated with having a handicapping condition and academic, behavioral and social competence enhancement (Galloway & Chandler, 1978; Blacher-Dixon et al., 1981). Through observational learning and direct educational experiences, the exceptional child may acquire academic, social, and behavioral skills from peers who stimulate, model, and reinforce their exceptional peers during interactions (Guralnick, 1981).

2) Societal acceptance of handicaps should be fostered through early exposure to exceptional children during the formative years of the children's development (Galloway & Chandler, 1978). This formative period coincides with the years during which children are involved in day-care and early childhood programs.

3) Program individualization as an educational goal can be actualized through the integration process, particularly in the context of early childhood programs (Guralnick, 1976). The instructional staff should be able to explore alternative curriculum materials and instructional strategies, thereby enhancing their instructional repertoire (Bricker & Sandall, 1979).

4) Integration should function as a preventive educational option; that is, segregated early placement often has negative iatrogenic side effects associated with the child's learning experiences. By initiating learning experiences within a typical preschool environment, many of these iatrogenic phenomena should be prevented or avoided.

5) Many special education planners assume that placement within

integrated settings will result in less expensive early educational costs for the child with special needs. Even with additional support staff, such as an itinerant teacher, the use of the natural environment in terms of classrooms, playgrounds, materials, and so on, may end up being less expensive than the provision of specialized segregated services.

The interaction literature suggests that although in vivo social interaction patterns are limited between exceptional and typical preschoolers (Feitelson, Weintraub, & Michaeli, 1972), several successful approaches are available to enhance and maintain the play and social interactions of children within integrated environments (Gresham, 1981; Snyder, Apolloni, & Cooke, 1977). Attention needs to be focused, however, upon the social validity of increases in social competence in the integrated setting, the maintenance of therapeutically induced changes, the spin-off on the nonhandicapped children's interaction patterns, and which methods may work for which handicapping conditions.

Research on nonhandicapped children's attitudes towards the handicapped suggests that early proximity and social interaction may lead to more positive views of the exceptional child (Corman & Gottlieb, 1978). However, much is yet to be clarified regarding the measurement of attitudes, early formation of attitudes, and the relationship between these beliefs and subsequent behavior patterns (Guralnick, 1981).

With regard to program characteristics, the teaching staff in preschool programs seem to provide a critical touchstone for the success of integrated programs. The presence of more favorable teacher attitudes toward integration during these early years (Larrivee & Cook, 1979) and the application of a "developmental competence" model (Garwood, 1979) to both Early Childhood and Special Education programs provide the unifying conceptual basis for the teacher's input into the program. Specialized skills and competencies would certainly be required by the integrated program teaching staff (Meisels, 1977). However, many teachers feel unprepared and, indeed, negative toward teaching within an integrated program (Childs, 1981). Hence, there is certainly a need for the provision of these competencies at the preservice or inservice levels of staff preparation.

A second major program feature is the type of program and the model of curriculum employed. As mentioned previously, the developmental competence notion certainly bridges one gap potentially separating Early Childhood and Special Education programs. Developmental and behavioral competencies or survival skills have been proposed by McDavid and Garwood (1978) which could provide the basis for assessing the exceptional child and subsequently planning and implementing an integrative intervention program.

Family involvement through integrated programs has been supported by researchers for many years (Bronfenbrenner, 1974; Honig, 1975; Zigler & Valentine, 1979). Families have been involved in particular because of their role in generalizing and maintaining competency-acquisition by their child (Karnes, 1979) as well as more generally building a strong attitudinal support for integration and service provision to their child (Allen, 1980; Blacher-Dixon et al., 1981). However, little research has systematically involved the family in the context of the preschool program and investigated parental input into the therapeutic process for the child.

Summary

Although research literature highlights some findings regarding the interaction patterns of students, attitudes of students and teachers, and limited suggestions regarding program development and implementation, many issues are unresolved or simply uninvestigated. Screening and diagnostic processes have yet to be clarified so that early integrated therapeutic experiences could be provided to attenuate potential developmental delays. Few authors have dealt with the management of day-to-day interactions between peers (both handicapped and nonhandicapped) within the integrated preschool environment on a long-term basis. The literature then seems to imply the potential success of integration but little assistance is provided regarding systematic phases of the integration process which require analysis and action.

DECISION-MAKING MODEL FOR INTEGRATION

A model for planning and implementing the integration process is presented in Figure 1. The four phases delineated in the figure represent the critical information gathering and analysis procedures carried out to accomplish effective integration. Each phase will be reviewed successively to describe the process in detail.

Information Gathering—Phase I

In Phase I, information regarding the child and family is obtained from at least four sources. First, a functional skills assessment is de-

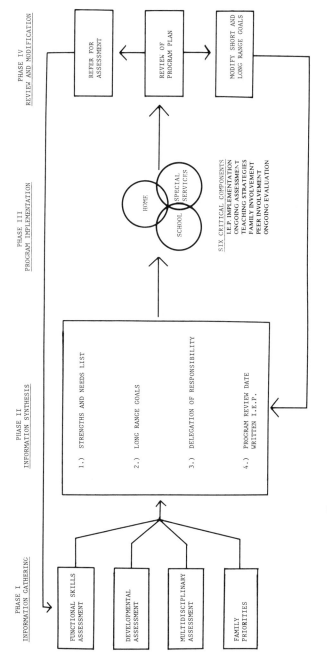

FIGURE 1. A model for planning and implementing the integration process

veloped for the current and future environments in which the child will be living (Brown, Branston-McClean, Baumgart, Vincent, Falvey, & Schroeder, 1979). Typically, the competencies measured in a functional skills assessment are extracted from the characteristics of the child's current and future environments whether they are domestic, educational, recreational, or community. For example, the preschool environment might yield several important activities (i.e., cooperative play) which require specific functional skills (e.g., sharing, conversation, requesting items) that the child should be learning within the integrated program. This method of assessment will also be utilized in an ongoing manner during the program implementation phase. At this initial phase of information gathering however, a positive medium for parental participation is provided (through an analysis of home and community environments) in preparation for the case conference or Individual Education Plan (I.E.P.) meeting.

Second, developmental assessments are required to determine developmental functioning and to assist in the decision regarding appropriate program placement. This developmental assessment (emphasizing such devices as the McCarthy Scales, 1972), should cover several areas of development and should subsequently assist in program planning.

Third, information gathering includes the multidisciplinary assessments required to specify any particular needs the child may have (speech therapy, physiotherapy, or medical needs, for example). The professional providing these data may also provide an ongoing special service to the child or family during program implementation.

Fourth, families' priorities and characteristics are assessed to establish a clear avenue of parent participation; this process would include an analysis of the home environment as well (Caldwell & Bradley, 1979) to determine the extent and type of family support. With some families it may be necessary to provide additional supportive services to assist the child's development and growth. The family's values and attitudes regarding the child's development and handicapping condition(s) will be essential input into the program planning process.

Information Synthesis—Phase II

In the second phase of the program development process the I.E.P. planning session will bring together the relevant persons (day-care or kindergarten staff, family members, specialists, and relevant others) to identify the child's strengths and needs, establish long-range goals, determine program implementation responsibility, and establish a time line for reviewing the child's placement. This information synthesis phase incorporates the development of the I.E.P. as the major method of information synthesis and program planning. The program planning phase provides for parents' participation in decision making and stresses the child's strengths as well as describing the child's special needs.

For the preschool program, this phase ensures the delineation of the purpose and direction of intervention and outlines who is responsible for what, by what date, with what resources, and under whose authority (thereby establishing the agent of accountability). This process should thus clarify the agency's responsibilities and the specific direction of assistance to both the child and family. The I.E.P. itself provides a written commitment of resources necessary to meet the child's special needs; it also provides for a monitoring device to ensure the provision of appropriate services which were mutually agreed upon by the constituents.

Within the I.E.P. itself, the specific special programs and related special services are typically stated, including a description of the scope and intensity of these therapeutic efforts; e.g., speech therapy, language therapy or physiotherapy. The extent and intensity of the exceptional child's participation within integrated program settings is also specified, at least initially, to ensure attention to social, academic, and cognitive development within the integrated, "least restrictive" environment. If possible, objective criteria and educational procedures are stated to serve as the bases for deciding upon the achievement of short-term and long-range goals.

Development of strengths and needs list. The provision of a strengths and needs list usually includes the educational, domestic, recreational, general community, health, and family domains. Often, cross-referencing between functional skills and developmental areas can assist the production of a strengths/needs list. For example, cognitive problem-solving competencies and toy manipulation can be strengths or needs in the cognitive development area but also be considered as activities or skills within the educational domain. Because these skills may also be functional within other domains, this list may provide the initial perspective for cross-domain or cross-situational program planning and generalization.

The strengths usually include a description of the individual's abilities and attempt to show direction for the matching of programs and activities to the individual's interests and preferences. This direction, for the young child, could include types of toys, play activities, preferred environments or persons, or modes of interaction.

The child's needs (and delays if appropriate) could be listed in each domain. This process would specify the areas in which the child requires assistance in developing competencies and/or changing patterns of behavior. Statements of need could indicate what the child needs to learn, do, increase, or expand and are typically stated positively. The child's developmental and special service needs would also be included in the needs list.

A primary goal of this activity is to provide as complete a profile as possible of the child's strengths and needs. Even though there may be considerable overlap, the unique perspectives presented by each I.E.P. conference team member will provide information of which other members may not have been aware. This list forms the basis for specific long-range goal statements.

Long range goals. Long-range goals are typically distilled from the specific needs list. Long-range goals are therefore reflections of the prioritization process of the child's needs by the conference team and include goals which the child will be moving towards during the next 10 to 12 months.

The goals themselves include exact descriptions of desired end behaviors or outcomes, usually with some statement of any special services which may be needed. The direction of desired change (increase, decrease, or maintain), the domain or developmental area and environments each may be described. The expected functioning level or status to be achieved when the goal is met will also form a part of the goal statement. For example, the following statement constitutes one long-range goal: "The learner will walk a minimum of 20 steps independently (Special Service: physiotherapy)." The concept here involves prioritization of needs into goals by the conference members, decisions regarding specific developmental areas and environments, and a decision delineating the expected time course of change (20 steps within x days/weeks/months). This allows evaluation of goal attainment to be made at intervals during the child's progress in the program.

Delegation of responsibility. Once the long-term goals have been established, each appropriate team member will take on responsibility for the implementation and monitoring of each long-range goal. In many instances it is obvious who will be responsible for particular long-range goals; e.g., the pediatrician can manage medication schedules. However, it may be necessary to assign more than one person to a goal; e.g., both the teacher and parent may be involved in the planning and implementation of a self-help or expressive language program. A tentative initiation date is also set at this time.

The person designated as responsible for the goal is required to devise the learning/instructional program or obtain the special services necessary to achieve the goal. The program planning process involves the analysis of long-range goals into sequenced instructional objectives, devising appropriate educational strategies, and establishing a specific evaluation procedure.

*Program review date and written I.E.P.*The final tasks of the I.E.P. conference include setting a date for review of the program and the completion and distribution of the written I.E.P. to all participants. Even though in special education it is common practice to communicate orally between team members (Yoshida, Fenton, Maxwell, & Kaufman, 1978), this type of communication can have a negative impact upon the clarity and consistency with which program plans are implemented. A written report also provides a permanent record for cross-referral, review, and subsequent evaluation.

Several researchers have found that interdisciplinary teams often experience difficulties with procedures for establishing goals and priorities, members' awareness of official objectives, interpersonal relationships, and role perceptions (Allen, Holm, & Schiefelbusch, 1978; Fenton, Yoshida, Maxwell, & Kaufman, 1979; Yoshida et al., 1978). Hopefully, safeguards such as those described in this section will reduce or prevent the emergence of these interfering factors in program development for the child.

Program Implementation—Phase III

The third phase of the decision-making process initiates programming for the child within the context of the long-range goals developed during the I.E.P. conference. As Figure 1 portrays, six critical components have been identified and require specific attention. Each component will be reviewed according to its various characteristics which require decisions.

Individual Education Program implementation. The long-range goals lead to specific short-term objectives for the purpose of establishing teaching/learning experiences within the integrated environment. Short-term objectives are small steps or components which lead to the attainment of long-term goals. These teaching objectives typically are specific, observable, measurable, compatible with client/family needs and agency objectives, and attainable by the child. Typically, these instructional objectives specify an observable behavior (performance) or product, describe the situation(s) within which the child will use the skill or competency, indicate the relevant conditions (e.g., time parameter, material), and specify accuracy, speed, or qualitative performance criteria (Baine, 1981). An example follows:

> Given five wooden blocks, 2″ × 2″ in size, the learner will stack five blocks to form an independently standing tower within one minute of task command. The learner will build a tower on a minimum of two of three trials for three consecutive days.

Depending upon the long-term goals, short-term objectives are derived via task analysis (Baine, 1981) or from developmental or behavioral curricula already prepared (e.g., Vulpe, 1979). That is, if the long-range goal specifies an area of developmental competence, the short-term objectives may be drawn from developmental sequences or progressions found in the "normal" population and specified in several curricula (Mori & Neisworth, 1983). Alternatively, the long-range goal may coincide with major objectives in a specific behavioral curriculum series (e.g., Teaching-Research Curriculum Series, Fredericks, Riggs, Furey, Grove, Moore, McDonnell, Jordan, Hanson, Baldwin, & Wadlow, 1976).

Task analysis, which is sometimes necessary for complex goals, requires the teacher to precisely delineate the specific steps of an objective, or "what" is to be taught. Once the skill or objective has been determined, the process of task analysis requires the identification of both the specific behavioral components of the skill, as well as any necessary prerequisite behaviors. Finally, the components are sequenced into a hierarchy such that the simpler skills, lower in the hierarchy, facilitate the acquisition of more complex tasks (Resnick, Wang, & Kaplan, 1973). The end result is an organized and precisely defined sequence of sub-skills from which the instructional objective is developed.

After the objectives are specified, the staff or person responsible typically prepares a specific program plan or format. The components of the specific program include the long- and short-term objectives, the functional domain, if appropriate, the developmental area, and the specific teaching procedures. As well, other factors such as when the skill is to be taught/learned, how often, in what settings, with which materials and reinforcers, and the data collection procedure are given. Finally, the steps and procedures to ensure generalization and maintenance are given.

Ongoing assessment. Ongoing evaluation can be built into the specific plan through the monitoring of a data-collection process. Such a data-based analysis of teaching (White & Liberty, 1976) provides for substantial analytic information regarding program efficacy. More generally, however, program staff may find it necessary and most appropriate to repeat specific criterion-referenced assessment to identify new short-term goals (see previous section regarding short-term goal statements) or to reexamine the child's functional skills and competencies using the functional skills inventory described previously.

As the child attains a competency described in a specific teaching plan, reassessment or probes may be required to determine the next skill or level of competency (fluency) in order to be certain that it will be the appropriate teaching objective in the subsequent plan. This process ensures that the program is responsive to the child's developing competencies.

Teaching strategies. The "nuts and bolts" of the intervention plan are the specific teaching/learning strategies. Three types will be briefly reviewed in this section which vary along the dimensions of structure, person initiating the exchange, and degree of environmental (ecological) validity.

Direct teaching (Becker, Engelmann, & Thomas, 1975) methods are usually structured, adult-initiated interactions which have been employed to effect very rapid acquisition of specific skills, competencies, or knowledge (concepts) with young children (Allen, 1980; Kysela, Daly, Doxsey-Whitfield, Hillyard, McDonald, McDonald, & Taylor, 1979). Many exceptional children require highly structured direct instruction to facilitate the acquisition of developmental, functional, and academic skills (Martin, Murrell, Nicholson, & Tallman, 1975). The methods are highly systematic, often employing prompts, modeling, and physical guidance. These methods are often needed to complement day-care and kindergarten general routines and activities, particularly increasing as the child's skill deficiencies increase with more severe handicapping conditions.

Incidental teaching, on the other hand, is an approach in which teachers and/or parents can use naturally occurring interactions, usually child-initiated, to transmit new information or to give the child a chance to practice, develop, or generalize the use of skills/concepts learned through direct teaching. This method facilitates generalization within group interactions to encourage developmental integration with peers (Mori & Neisworth, 1983) through simultaneous teaching of several children at different functional levels. It allows the staff and parents to exploit "teachable moments" which occur during the child's day. While these strategies have often been used in language instruction (Hart & Risley, 1975; Hart & Rogers-Warren, 1978), a variety of other developmental competencies could be taught/learned in this manner: for example, self-help and motoric skills (Kysela et al., 1979).

The following steps are usually employed with incidental teaching. After child initiation, adult attention is the first cue showing expectation of further response/verbalization. If the child does not respond, a further verbal cue is provided; e.g., "What do you want?" If the child still does not respond, gestural or modeled cues can be provided, while for motoric responses (such as pointing, walking, etc.) physical guidance may be ultimately used to lead the child through the response (Kysela et al., 1979).

Ecological teaching strategies (MacDonald, 1982) combine characteristics of both of the preceding methods. These ecological strategies are either adult-initiated, as in the use of communication stations, or child-initiated within naturally arising opportunities for communicative interaction occurring throughout the day in school or home. These strategies have been developed to cover four developmental areas essential in language acquisition: social interaction/turn-taking conversations; language mode—nonverbal, vocal, words and phrases; content of child's communications; and functional use—personal, social, and instrumental purposes.

Strategies to facilitate social interaction include imitating the child, structuring interactions for turn taking and give-and-take, waiting for the child to respond, and signaling and prompting a response if the child does not take a turn. Strategies of modeling the correct responses and imitating and expanding the child's utterances or words are recommended as well (MacDonald, 1982). These strategies can be used spontaneously to nurture extended communication exchanges and interactions as well as to develop competencies in other developmental areas.

Peer involvement. Support for integrated programs has been argued on the basis that such programs provide opportunity for the handicapped to profit from both indirect (by observing models of more developmentally sophisticated behavior) and direct contact (through verbal and nonverbal social interaction) with nonhandicapped peers (Apolloni & Cooke, 1975; Bricker, 1978). However, research appears to indicate that in the absence of intervention, a lack of interaction between two groups is generally the rule (Guralnick, 1980; Peterson & Haralick, 1977) and spontaneous imitation of peer models by the handicapped is rare (Guralnick, 1976; Snyder et al., 1977). It would appear that physical integration of the handicapped is a necessary, but not sufficient condition for cross-group interaction (Rogers-Warren, 1982).

In the last two decades, a wide variety of strategies have been developed in an attempt to facilitate the development and maintenance of peer interaction and/or imitative behaviors. Researchers have investigated such procedures as contingent adult attention (e.g., Apolloni & Cooke, 1975), token systems (e.g., Knapczyk & Yoppi, 1975), symbolic modeling (Gottman, 1977), coaching and behavioral rehearsal (Ladd, 1981) as well as manipulation of the physical, spatial, and organizational features of the classroom setting (Strain, 1975) to facilitate peer interaction.

Recently, there has been increased interest in the role of nonhandicapped peers effecting change in the social behavior of their withdrawn classmates. It has been demonstrated that few of the adult-mediated techniques produce generalized behavior change outside the treatment setting (Strain & Hill, 1979). As well, implementation of such procedures assumes that the teacher is well trained in the principles of behavior modification and able to correctly implement the procedures. Considering the number of children who are identified as in need of intervention, it is unlikely that an adult-mediated strategy is a practical option in most preschool programs.

Secondly, an analysis of the immediate temporal effects of adult reinforcement indicates that contingent adult attention served to terminate the ongoing interactions between handicapped and nonhandicapped children (Strain & Hill, 1979). While the frequency of discrete social behaviors was dramatically increased, the resulting interactions were very brief and artificial, "similar to cocktail party or table-hopping behavior" (Hops, Walker, & Greenwood, 1977, p. 12). These procedures have not been successful in developing and/or maintaining the extended interaction episodes which are characteristic of socially competent children (Strain & Fox, 1981). Finally, evidence from naturalistic-observational (Guralnick & Paul-Brown, 1977) and intervention studies (Wahler, 1967) clearly indicated that peer contingencies had a significant impact on the development and maintenance of peer interactions.

A wide variety of peer-mediated strategies (i.e., modeling, prompting and reinforcement, social initiations) have been developed in the last decade. For example, Strain and his colleagues have conducted a series of studies investigating the functional effects of an increased rate of social initiations by nonhandicapped children on the social behavior of handicapped children (Strain & Fox, 1981). It was demonstrated that the onset of peer social initiations produced an immediate increase in positive social behavior in most subjects. However, children exhibiting a lower baseline level of social behavior were less responsive to the treatment than children with higher baseline performances (Strain, Kerr, & Ragland, 1979).

Family involvement. Parent/family involvement in the education of preschool handicapped children is considered to be a critical element in the success of integrated programs (Baker, 1976; Calvert, 1971). The involvement of parents in the assessment process allows them to function more effectively as part of the team during the second phase of the program-planning process, during which program priorities and long-range goals are established. While parents are often accused of having unrealistic expectations for their children, such behavior is not surprising when parents are not familiar with, or part of, the assessment process. It is also believed that parents who are actively involved in long-range goal setting are more likely to support and therefore implement the programs designed to achieve those goals (Vincent, Brown, & Getz-Sheftel, 1981).

The involvement of parents in the third phase of the process, program implementation, is supported by research which clearly indicates greater child progress when parents were actively involved (Bricker & Sandall, 1979; Hanson, 1977). The lack of skill generalization and maintenance by handicapped students (Stokes & Baer, 1977) has prompted educators to acknowledge that programming must be extended outside the classroom setting. Simultaneous home/school instruction has been shown to accelerate the rate of acquisition of some skills (Fredericks, Baldwin, & Grove, 1976), and it is also possible that some skills, such as self-help, can be more appropriately taught at home, thereby freeing school time for other tasks. Parents have been successfully trained to use behavior management strategies and various instructional strategies to develop cognitive, communication, motor, social, and self-help skills (Baker, 1976; Feldman, Byalick, & Rosedale, 1975; Kysela et al., 1979). For young children, parents are also a natural and powerful source of reinforcement, and can therefore have a significant impact on the child's achievement of instructional objectives (Kelley, Embry, & Baer, 1979; Tharp & Wetzel, 1969). In fact, it has been reported that trained parents are able to elicit more responsiveness from their children than professionals (Schopler & Reichler, 1971).

Acquisition of programming skills has reportedly enhanced the parents' perceptions of their ability to cope with their child, decreased reports of frustration and highlighted their ability to significantly affect their child's development (Feldman et al., 1975). Parents also reported that training made them more capable of evaluating the quality and appropriateness of the educational services that their child was receiving (Baker, 1976), which would make them more effective advocates for the child in the final review and modification phase of the planning process.

Ongoing evaluation. Most programs integrating handicapped or exceptional children within "typical" preschool environments provide for systematic evaluation during the program to "trouble-shoot" any arising difficulties and to provide feedback regarding the child's progress in order to adjust or redevelop teaching plans and strategies. Such ongoing evaluation should provide continuous monitoring on a regular basis of the child's progress in each curriculum area in which teaching plans are being implemented (Bricker & Sandall, 1979).

Ongoing data collection in the teaching plan provides one method of evaluating specific progress. The traditional educational practice of assessing the child's progress at widely spaced intervals, often with normative, standardized measures, does not provide the teacher with sufficient information to judge the effectiveness of the individual educational plan. However, the ongoing evaluation of data obtained from the program on a daily or weekly basis will be extremely useful to decide upon teaching plan changes and revisions.

A second type of ongoing evaluation builds into the treatment regimen a research design to yield either process evaluation or outcome data. The use of applied behavior analysis designs such as reversals or multiple baseline (Hersen & Barlow, 1976), changing criterion designs (Hartmann & Hall, 1976), and other time series designs (Kratochwill, 1978) as an integral dimension of the teaching plan will provide systematic analytic data regarding the specific effects of programs.

The use of criterion-referenced assessment devices, as described in the sections on assessment, can be employed to assist in child progress evaluation. That is, as the child moves through various phases of instructional programs the repeated use of criterion-referenced measures allows the staff to observe and share with others independent measures of the child's increasing behavioral competency (Bricker & Dow, 1980). In addition, developmental assessments could be employed to similarly mark any increasing developmental competence the child exhibits (Garwood, 1979).

Finally, frequent contact with parents and significant others in the child's life provides a basis for determining the social validity of success of intervention and the integration process. These ongoing measures may include parental ratings and interviews, measures of social/cognitive development, language development and personal adjustment, peer ratings of social acceptability and attitudes towards the handicapped, and staff satisfaction with the program's impact upon the child, peers, and school.

In summary, then, each of these six critical components provides a step in the process of implementing an integrated individual educational plan for the exceptional child. Attention to these parameters should reduce the risk of attrition often found when moderately to severely handicapped young children are integrated into regular school settings.

Program Review and Modification—Phase IV

In the fourth phase of the integration process, program review and appropriate modification are considered. As Figure 1 portrays, two major feedback loops exist from Phase IV back to reassessment in Phase I or to Phase II and Phase III for revision of the I.E.P. and implementation of new teaching/learning plans.

In this fourth phase, the decision-making process exhibits a responsiveness to changes in the child's developmental competencies, skills, knowledge, and needs. Hence, in addition to the ongoing evaluation of the child's progress in specific teaching plans, mentioned previously, arrangements should be made for the entire I.E.P. conference team to periodically review the total educational plan. At this time, adjustments can be made to the long-range goals or to the priorities assigned to existing goals. Specific short-range objectives and teaching strategies may also be modified, withdrawn, or added to meet newly arising needs.

Referrals for reassessment of specific facets of the child's functional skills and knowledge, developmental status, and physical/sensory functions may also be necessary from time to time. Shifting family priorities may require a realignment of program priorities for the child as well. The review and modification processes of this phase ensure the relevancy of the educational plans and activities to the child's current and future needs.

Thus, as far as possible, the design of the decision-making model and the individualized planning/intervention process are associated with the attempt to maximize the positive impact of integration upon the child's educational, community, and domestic experiences. At the same time, the demands of the planning process upon the significant participants are minimized. Overly complex and time-consuming procedures could adversely interfere with the efficiency and effectiveness of the participants while a superficial and hasty planning process may produce minimal benefits to the child.

PERSONNEL PREPARATION

In this final section, issues regarding the professional preparation of staff (child care workers, rehabilitation specialists, and teachers) for integrated programs will be considered. Several authors investigating the integration process have stressed the importance of preparing the teaching and program staff in the development of specific skills and competencies necessary to manage an integrated setting (Allen, 1980; Raver, 1980; Zigler & Muenchow, 1979). In fact, Turnbull, Strickland, and Hammer (1978) have suggested that without adequate personnel preparation, the I.E.P. can be dismissed as an impossible educational alternative.

Several studies have found that "mainstreaming" teachers often feel a lack of skills and competencies to integrate handicapped children into their classrooms (Baker & Gottlieb, 1980; Shotel, Iano, & McGettigan, 1972). In the absence of support services and inservice, Shotel et al. (1972) also demonstrated a substantial *drop* in teachers' estimates of their competency in working with handicapped children over the course of a school year. Since relatively few regular class teachers have special education training (Baker & Gottlieb, 1980), it seems that this problem will persist.

Given the apparent need to provide appropriate specific training to those working with the exceptional child, this decision-making model can be seen to serve two purposes: *First,* the model can be used to ensure a thorough planning and implementation process for the integration of an exceptional child into the preschool environment; *second,* it can serve as a guide for staff to judge their own skills and competencies. As the staff become familiar with the integration decision-making model and attendant processes, they should be able to pinpoint the specific skills required to fulfill their role in each phase of the process. The staff members should then be able to judge where their strengths and weaknesses lie, and should delineate the scope and content of the specific inservice training required. Preservice training and experience of prospective staff members could also be assessed more clearly relative to specific job requirements.

Summary

The placement of exceptional children into "typical" or "least restrictive" preschool settings has become an increasingly popular educational alternative in the last decade. In the broadest sense, this practice can be viewed as a manifestation of the "normalization" principle (Wolfensberger, 1972) which asserts the right of the exceptional child to an appropriate education within a setting as close as possible to that offered normal children. Further, integration has been advocated on the basis of its supposed positive impact upon the exceptional child and his or her family, the normally developing peers and their families, the school personnel, as well as the community at large.

However, a review of the research literature available to date indicates that many of the purported benefits which have been claimed to be associated with integrated placements for exceptional children have not been entirely supported by direct empirical evidence. Indeed, it would appear that in the absence of systematic planning and personnel preparation, the mere physical placement of the exceptional child in a regular setting can produce effects entirely counterproductive to the goals of integration. Some attempts have been made to outline methods that can be used to ensure that these critical factors are incorporated into the program structure.

Given this ambiguity encountered in the current professional literature, it has been suggested that the proposed decision-making model can be used by those in applied settings to serve two functions. First, it can be seen as a process which guides practitioners through the planning and implementation of the integration model, while facilitating open, continuing communication between all the significant agents involved with the exceptional child. Further, systematically working through each of the four phases ensures the coverage of each facet necessary to accomplish effective integration: assessment, establishment of long-range goals, instructional program planning, program implementation, staff competencies, parental involvement, supportive services, program evaluation and accountability. However, it should be noted that little evaluative data are available examining the use of this model for program planning or implementation; such an analysis is essential to ultimately determine the model's usefulness and value.

Second, the model can serve as a guide which will enable staff members to pinpoint the skills and competencies needed to fulfill their roles in each phase of the decision-making process and, therefore, assist them to delineate more precisely their future training needs. The use of this model can ensure that the personnel working with the child are adequately prepared and more confident of their ability to deal effectively with the child's needs, as well as ensuring that all of the necessary steps have been taken to maximize the positive impact of integration upon the child's educational, home, and community experiences.

REFERENCES

ACKERMAN, P. R., & MOORE, M. G. (1976). Delivery of educational services to preschool handicapped children. In T. D. Tjossem (Ed.), *Intervention strategies for high-risk infants and young children*. Baltimore: University Park Press.

ALLEN, K. E. (1980). *Mainstreaming in early childhood education*. Albany, NY: Delmar Publishers.

ALLEN, K. E., HOLM, V. A., & SCHIEFELBUSCH, R. L. (Eds.). (1978). *Early intervention—A team approach*. Baltimore: University Park Press.

APOLLONI, T., & COOKE, T. P. (1975). Peer behavior conceptualized as a variable influencing infant and toddler development. *American Journal of Orthopsychiatry, 45*, 4-17.

BAINE, D. (1981). *Instructional design for special education*. Englewood Cliffs, NJ: Educational Technology Publications.

BAKER, B. L. (1976). Parent involvement in programming for developmentally disabled children. In L. L. Lloyd (Ed.), *Communication assessment and intervention strategies*. Baltimore: University Park Press.

BAKER, J. L., & GOTTLIEB, J. (1980). Attitudes of teachers towards mainstreaming retarded children. In J. Gottlieb (Ed.), *Educating mentally retarded persons in the mainstream*. Baltimore: University Park Press.

BECKER, W. C., ENGELMANN, S., & THOMAS, D. R. (1975). *Teaching 2: Cognitive learning and instruction*. Toronto: Science Research Associates.

BLACHER-DIXON, J., LEONARD, J., & TURNBULL, A. P. (1981). Mainstreaming at the early childhood level: Current and future perspectives. *Mental Retardation, 19*, 235-241.

BRICKER, D. D. (1978). A rationale for the integration of handicapped and nonhandicapped preschool children. In M. J. Guralnick (Ed.), *Early intervention and the integration of handicapped children*. Baltimore: University Park Press.

BRICKER, D. D., & DOW, M. (1980). Early intervention with the young severely handicapped child. *Journal of the Association for the Severely Handicapped, 5*, 130-142.

BRICKER, D., & SANDALL, S. (1979). Mainstreaming in preschool programs: How and why to do it. *Education Unlimited, 1*, 25-29.

BRONFENBRENNER, U. (1974). *Is early intervention effective?* Washington, DC: Department of Health, Education and Welfare, Publication No. 74-25.

BROWN, L., BRANSTON-MCCLEAN, M. B., BAUMGART, D., VINCENT, L., FALVEY, M., & SCHROEDER, J. (1979). Using the characteristics of current and subsequent least restrictive environments in the development of curricula content for severely handicapped students. *AAESPH Review, 4*, 407-424.

CALDWELL, B. M., & BRADLEY, R. H. (1979). *Home observation for measurement of the environment*. Little Rock, AR: Center for Child Development and Education, University of Arkansas.

CALVERT, D. R. (1971). Dimensions of family involvement in early childhood education. *Exceptional Children, 37*, 655-659.

CARLBERG, C., & KOVALE, K. (1980). The efficacy of special versus regular class placement for exceptional children: A meta-analysis. *The Journal of Special Education, 14*, 295-309.

CHILDS, R. E. (1981). Perceptions of mainstreaming by regular classroom teachers who teach educable mentally retarded students in the public schools. *Education and Training of the Mentally Retarded, 16*, 325-327.

CORMAN, L., & GOTTLIEB, J. (1978). Mainstreaming mentally retarded children: A review of research. In N. R. Ellis (Ed.), *International review of research in mental retardation* (Vol. 9). New York: Academic Press.

DUNN, L. M. (1968). Special education for the mildly retarded—Is much of it justifiable? *Exceptional Children, 23*, 5-22.

FEITELSON, D., WEINTRAUB, S., & MICHAELI, O. (1972). Social interaction in heterogeneous preschools in Israel. *Child Development, 43*, 1249-1259.

FELDMAN, M. A., BYALICK, R., & ROSEDALE, M. P. (1975). Parent involvement programs: A growing trend in special education. *Exceptional Children, 41*, 356-358.

FENTON, K. S., YOSHIDA, R. K., MAXWELL, J. P., & KAUFMAN, M. J. (1979). Recognition of team goals: An essential step toward rational decision making. *Exceptional Children, 45*, 638-644.

FREDERICKS, H. D., RIGGS, C., FUREY, T., GROVE, D., MOORE, W., MCDONNELL, J., JORDAN, E., HANSON, W., BALDWIN, V., & WADLOW, M. (1976). *The teaching research curriculum for moderately and severely handicapped*. Springfield, IL: Charles C Thomas.

FREDERICKS, D., BALDWIN, V. L., & GROVE, D. A. (1976). A home-center-based parent-training model. In D. L. Lillie, P. L. Trohanis, & K. W. Goin (Eds.), *Teaching parents to teach: A guide for working with the special child*. New York: Walker.

GALLOWAY, C., & CHANDLER, P. (1978). The marriage of special and generic early education services. In M. J. Guralnick (Ed.), *Early intervention and the integration of handicapped and nonhandicapped children*. Baltimore: University Park Press.

GARWOOD, S. G. (1979). *Educating young handicapped children: A developmental approach.* Germantown, MD: Aspen Systems.

GOTTMAN, J. (1977). The effects of a modeling film on social isolation in preschool children: A methodological investigation. *Journal of Abnormal Child Psychology, 5,* 69-78.

GRESHAM, F. M. (1981). Social skills training with handicapped children: A review. *Review of Educational Research, 51,* 139-176.

GURALNICK, M. J. (1976). The value of integrating handicapped and nonhandicapped preschool children. *American Journal of Orthopsychiatry, 41,* 236-245.

GURALNICK, M. J. (1980). Social interactions among preschool children. *Exceptional Children, 46,* 248-253.

GURALNICK, M. J. (1981). Peer influences on the development of communicative competence. In P. S. Strain (Ed.), *The utilization of classroom peers as behavior change agents.* New York: Plenum Press.

GURALNICK, M. J., & PAUL-BROWN, D. (1977). The nature of verbal interactions among handicapped and nonhandicapped preschool children. *Child Development, 48,* 254-260.

HANSON, M. (1977). *Teaching your Down's Syndrome infant: A guide for parents.* Baltimore: University Park Press.

HART, B., & RISLEY, T. R. (1975). Incidental teaching of language in the preschool. *Journal of Applied Behavior Analysis, 8,* 411-420.

HART, B., & ROGERS-WARREN, A. G. (1978). A milieu approach to teaching language. In R. L. Schiefelbusch (Ed.), *Language intervention strategies.* Baltimore: University Park Press.

HARTMANN, D. P., & HALL, R. V. (1976). The changing criterion design. *Journal of Applied Behavior Analysis, 9,* 527-532.

HERSEN, M., & BARLOW, D. H. (1976). *Single-case experimental designs: Strategies for studying behavior change.* New York: Pergamon Press.

HONIG, A. (1975). *Parent involvement in early childhood education.* Washington, DC: National Association for the Education of Young Children.

HOPS, H., WALKER, H. M., & GREENWOOD, C. R. (1977). *PEERS—A program for remediating social withdrawal in the school setting: Aspects of a research and development process.* Eugene, OR: Center at Oregon for Research in the Behavioral Education of the Handicapped.

KARNES, M. B. (1979). The use of volunteers and parents in mainstreaming. *Viewpoints in Teaching and Learning, 55,* 44-56.

KAUFMAN, M. J., GOTTLIEB, J., AGARD, J. S., & KUKIC, M. B. (1975). Mainstreaming: Towards an explanation of the construct. In E. L. Meyer, G. A. Vergason, & R. J. Whelan (Eds.), *Alternatives for teaching exceptional children.* Denver: Love Publishing.

KELLEY, M. L., EMBRY, L. H., & BAER, D. M. (1979). Skills for child management and family support: Training parents for maintenance. *Behavior Modification, 3,* 373-396.

KNAPCZYK, D. R., & YOPPI, J. (1975). Development of cooperative and competitive play response in developmentally disabled children. *American Journal of Mental Deficiency, 80,* 245-255.

KRATOCHWILL, T. R. (1978). Foundations of time-series research. In T. R. Kratochwill (Ed.), *Single subject research: Strategies for evaluating change.* New York: Academic Press.

KYSELA, G. M., DALY, K. DOXSEY-WHITFIELD, M., HILLYARD, A., McDONALD, L., McDONALD, S., & TAYLOR, J. (1979). The early education project. In L. A. Hamerlynck (Ed.), *Behavioral systems for the developmentally disabled: I. School and family environments.* New York: Brunner/Mazel.

LADD, G. W. (1981). Effectiveness of a social learning method for enhancing children's social interaction and peer acceptance. *Child Development, 51,* 171-178.

LARRIVEE, B., & COOK, L. (1979). Mainstreaming: A study of variables affecting teacher attitude. *Journal of Special Education, 13*, 315-324.

MACDONALD, J. (1982). Language through conversation: A communicative model for language intervention. In S. Warren & A. G. Rogers-Warren (Eds.), *Productive language teaching*. Baltimore: University Park Press.

MARTIN, G., MURRELL, M., NICHOLSON, C., & TALLMAN, B. (1975). *Teaching basic skills to the severely and profoundly retarded: The MIMR basic behavior test, curriculum guide and programming strategy*. Portage La Prairie, Manitoba: Vopii Press.

MCCARTHY, D. (1972). *Manual for the McCarthy scale of children's abilities*. New York: The Psychological Corporation.

MCDAVID, J. W., & GARWOOD, S. G. (1978). *Understanding children*. Lexington, MA: D. C. Heath.

MEISELS, S. J. (1977). First steps in mainstreaming: Some questions and answers. *Young Children, 33*, 4-13.

MORI, A. A., & NEISWORTH, J. T. (1983). Curricula in early childhood education: Some generic and special considerations. *Topics in Early Childhood Special Education, 2*(4), 1-8.

PETERSON, N. L., & HARALICK, J. G. (1977). Integration of handicapped and nonhandicapped preschoolers: An analysis of play behavior and social interaction. *Education and Training of the Mentally Retarded, 12*, 235-245.

RAVER, S. A. (1980). Ten rules for success in preschool mainstreaming. *Education Unlimited, 2*, 47-52.

RESNICK, L., WANG, M., & KAPLAN, J. (1973). Task analysis in curriculum design: A hierarchically sequenced introductory mathematics curriculum. *Journal of Applied Behavior Analysis, 6*, 679-710.

ROGERS-WARREN, A. K. (1982). Behavioral ecology in classrooms for young, handicapped children. *Topics in Early Childhood Special Education, 2*(1), 21-32.

SAFFORD, P. L., & ROSEN, L. A. (1981). Mainstreaming: Application of a philosophical perspective in an integrated kindergarten program. *Topics in Early Childhood Special Education, 1*(1), 1-10.

SCHOPLER, E., & REICHLER, R. J. (1971). Parents as co-therapists in the treatment of psychotic children. *Journal of Autism and Childhood Schizophrenia, 1*, 87-102.

SHOTEL, J. R., IANO, R. P., & MCGETTIGAN, J. F. (1972). Teacher attitudes associated with the integration of handicapped children. *Exceptional Children, 38*, 677-683.

SNYDER, L., APOLLONI, T., & COOKE, T. P. (1977). Integrated settings at the early childhood level: The role of the nonretarded peers. *Exceptional Children, 43*, 262-266.

STOKES, T. F., & BAER, D. M. (1977). An implicit technology of generalization. *Journal of Applied Behavior Analysis, 10*, 349-367.

STRAIN, P. S. (1975). Increasing social play among severely mentally retarded preschool children with socio-dramatic activities. *Mental Retardation, 13*, 7-9.

STRAIN, P. S., & FOX, J. J. (1981). Peer social initiation and the modification of social withdrawal: A review and future perspectives. *Journal of Pediatric Psychology, 6*, 417-433.

STRAIN, P. S., & HILL, A. D. (1979). Social interaction training with the severely handicapped. In P. Wehman (Ed.), *Leisure time skills for the severely handicapped*. Baltimore: University Park Press.

STRAIN, P. S., KERR, M. M., & RAGLAND, E. U. (1979). Effects of peer mediated social initiations and prompting/reinforcement procedures on the social behavior of autistic children. *Journal of Autism and Developmental Disorders, 9*, 41-54.

TELFORD, C. W., & SAWREY, J. M. (1981). *The exceptional individual* (4th ed.). Englewood Cliffs, NJ: Prentice-Hall.

THARP, R. G., & WETZEL, R. J. (1969). *Behavior modification in the natural environment*. New York: Academic Press.

TURNBULL, A. P., STRICKLAND, B., & HAMMER, S. E. (1978). The individualized education program—Part 2: Translating law into practice. *Journal of Learning Disabilities, 11,* 18-23.

VINCENT, L. J., BROWN, L., & GETZ-SHEFTEL, M. (1981). Integrating the handicapped and typical children during the preschool years: The definition of best educational practice. *Topics in Early Childhood Special Education, 1*(1), 17-24.

VULPE, S. G. (1979). *Vulpe assessment battery* (2nd ed.). Toronto: National Institute on Mental Retardation.

WAHLER, R. G. (1967). Child-child interactions in free field settings: Some experimental analyses. *Journal of Experimental Child Psychology, 5,* 278-298.

WHITE, O., & LIBERTY, K. (1976). Behavioral assessment and precise educational measurement. In N. G. Haring & R. L. Schiefelbusch (Eds.), *Teaching special children.* New York: McGraw-Hill.

WILTON, K., & DENSEM, P. (1977). Social interaction of intellectually handicapped children in integrated and segregated preschools. *Exceptional Child, 24,* 165-172.

WOLFENSBERGER, W. (1972). *Normalization in human services.* Toronto: National Institute on Mental Retardation.

YOSHIDA, R. K., FENTON, K.S., MAXWELL, J. P., & KAUFMAN, M. J. (1978). Ripple effect: Communication of planning team decisions to program implementers. *Journal of School Psychology, 16,* 177-183.

ZIGLER, E. & MUENCHOW, S. (1979). Mainstreaming: The proof is in the implementation. *American Psychologist, 34,* 993-996.

ZIGLER, E., & VALENTINE, J. (Eds.). (1979). *Project Head Start: A legacy of the war on poverty.* New York: Free Press.

7

Social Skills Training in School Settings: A Model for the Social Integration of Handicapped Children Into Less Restrictive Settings

HILL M. WALKER, SCOTT R. MCCONNELL,
and JAMES Y. CLARKE

With the passage of Public Law 94-142, increasing numbers of mildly, moderately, and, in some cases, severely handicapped children are receiving at least part of their daily instruction in mainstream settings; e.g., regular classrooms and playgrounds. It was assumed by the framers and advocates of this law that the normalizing processes and developmental opportunities resulting from exposure to less restrictive settings would more than offset any deleterious effects associated with such placement. At present, sufficient data and follow-up studies do not exist to provide an unequivocal basis for accepting or rejecting this hypothesis. However, the social-behavioral adjustment of mainstreamed handicapped children is a topic of increasing professional concern to educators (e.g., Asher & Taylor, 1981).

When young children first enter preschool or regular school settings, they are required to make two major social-behavioral adjustments

(Walker, McConnell, Walker, Clarke, Todis, Cohen, & Rankin, 1983). That is, they must simultaneously adjust to the demands of the school setting *and* to a new peer group that is likely to be more demographically heterogeneous than any encountered within previous, nonschool environments. The adequacy with which these adjustments are made charts both the progress and direction of the child's long-term academic and social development (Brophy & Good, 1970; Robins, 1966).

The complexity and magnitude of these adjustments are frequently underestimated by parents, teachers, and researchers. In most instances, adequate adjustments require elaborate networks of interrelated, prerequisite generic and setting-specific skills and the social perception necessary to guide appropriate response to a variety of social contexts and school settings. The skills and competencies necessary to cope effectively with school demands are quite different from those contributing to social competence in peer-to-peer relationships.

In the area of school setting demands, for example, the young child must 1) meet the behavioral expectations or standards established by the school and individual teachers, 2) learn to respond appropriately within an academic context, and 3) develop the ability to follow narrowly defined behavioral rules that exist across school settings (e.g., listening to teacher instructions, using free time appropriately, displaying appropriate group behavior, working on assigned tasks, following directions, and making assistance needs known appropriately). Evidence for the impact of adaptive classroom behavior on academic achievement has been well established both *correlationally* (Bloom, 1976; Hoge & Luce, 1979), and *experimentally* (Cobb & Hops, 1973; Greenwood, Hops, & Walker, 1977).

Of equal importance and, perhaps, greater complexity, are the demands and pressures placed upon a young child by a new and heterogeneous peer group. The young child, for example, must learn how to 1) develop friendships, 2) initiate and respond appropriately to peers, 3) join groups of children already engaged in an ongoing activity, 4) extend invitations, 5) sustain interactive sequences over time, 6) communicate effectively, and 7) detect and accommodate to changing behavioral standards across social contexts within free play settings (Gottman, Gonso, & Rasmussen, 1975; Greenwood, Walker, Todd, & Hops, 1981; Guralnick, 1981). Many children do not have the socialization opportunities to develop this complex array of skills. This is especially true of young handicapped children.

It seems clear that many *nonhandicapped* school children are inadequately prepared to make the major adjustments required of them upon entry into the school setting (Asher & Gottman, 1981). Handicapped children, on the other hand, consistently show deficiencies in the critical skills required for successful adjustment to the demands of the school setting and those of a new peer group (Greenwood et al., 1981; Gresham, 1981, 1982; Hartup, 1979).

Normal children demonstrate substantial variability in their ability to appropriately display the critically important behavioral competencies (Greenwood, Todd, Hops, & Walker, 1982; Greenwood, Walker, Todd, & Hops, 1979; Hops & Finch, 1981) that underlie adjustment capability in school and peer-group settings. In addition, low interacting children typically initiate less, respond less frequently to peers' initiations to them, and are less verbal (Greenwood et al., 1982). Socially unpopular children also demonstrate deficiencies in a variety of key social competencies, such as cooperation and effective communication of their needs (Gottman et al., 1975; Oden & Asher, 1977). Handicapped children are highly likely to have low levels of social participation with peers in school settings, and to not be accepted by them (see Gottlieb, 1978; Gresham, 1981, 1982).

The developmental implications of these findings are extremely serious for both nonhandicapped and handicapped children. The available evidence suggests that children who are unable to make these crucial adjustments are at risk for both *school failure* and *serious developmental problems.*

The literature on teacher expectations and their behavioral expression (Brophy & Evertson, 1981; Brophy & Good, 1970) has been impressive in documenting the differential treatment of children for whom they hold high and low academic and behavioral expectations. In a now classic study, Brophy and Good (1970) showed that teachers behaved in ways toward high expectation students that tended to maximize their achievement (e.g., more cues, prompts, feedback, and praise for appropriate behavior). In contrast, they tended to minimize the achievement of low expectation students (e.g., fewer cues and prompts, less feedback and praise, and more criticism of their performance). Further, they were more likely to give up easily when dealing with low expectation students. Low expectation students, for most teachers, fall into disadvantaged, low socioeconomic status, and handicapped categories (Brophy & Evertson, 1981).

This evidence suggests that handicapped children placed in classroom settings where they fall below minimal teacher expectation levels may not be receiving the quality educational experience envisioned for them by Public Law 94-142. Research reviewed by Kornblau and Keogh

(1980) shows that teacher perceptions of the attributes or causes underlying deficient child performance can shape expectations and negatively affect teaching interactions. Handicapped children are particularly vulnerable to these processes.

The results of longitudinal and retrospective studies of children who are judged socially incompetent early in their school careers are even more devastating. Socially unskilled children have a high incidence of school maladjustment (Gronlund & Anderson, 1957), dropping out of school, and delinquency (Roff, Sells, & Golden, 1972), and bad conduct discharges from the military (Roff, 1961). Furthermore, peer status of elementary school students was highly predictive for mental health referrals up to 13 years later (Cowen, Pederson, Babigan, Izzo, & Trost, 1973). Other correlates of patterns of nonsocial behavior among young children include: 1) higher anxiety levels and less willingness to engage the environment, 2) submissiveness and variability in self-esteem, and 3) higher levels of anxiety and aggression (Bronson, 1966).

When one considers the evidence regarding the stability of children's maladaptive and deficient behavior patterns over time (Zax, Cowen, Rappaport, Beach, & Laird, 1968), it is unlikely that the mere passage of time, maturational processes, or the ordinary schooling experience will ameliorate child problems of this magnitude. Extraordinary measures are required to reduce the developmental risks of children who become highly visible because of either behavioral or social incompetence.

This chapter describes the development and initial validation of a model program designed to facilitate the social integration of handicapped children into less restrictive settings. The Social Behavior Survival (SBS) model program was developed via a 3-year Handicapped Children's Model Program grant to the senior author from the U.S. Office of Special Education Programs.

The remainder of this chapter is divided into three major sections. The first section presents information on the current knowledge base relating to the status of handicapped children in mainstream settings, and the technology governing the integration process. The second section describes the SBS model program and the development processes used in the assessment and intervention components of the model. The third section reports three experiments relating to the testing and revision of the ACCEPTS social skills training program (Walker, McConnell, Holmes, Todis, Walker, & Golden, 1983). ACCEPTS (**A** **C**urriculum for **C**hildren's **E**ffective **P**eer and **T**eacher **S**kills) is an instructional and behavior management program for teaching essential social skills required to achieve satisfactory social adjustment in less restrictive settings.

RESEARCH FINDINGS ON MAINSTREAMING AND
SOCIAL INTEGRATION INTO LESS RESTRICTIVE SETTINGS

The existing knowledge base relating to social skills and the mainstreaming process is reviewed in three areas: 1) research evidence on the status of mainstreamed handicapped children; 2) traditional approaches to least restrictive environment (LRE) placements in school settings; and 3) necessary conditions governing effective social integration into LRE school settings.

Research Evidence on the Status of Mainstreamed Handicapped Children

The available literature on teacher attitudes toward mainstreaming shows that 1) regular teachers are not as receptive toward it as we would perhaps like (Alexander & Strain, 1978; Keogh & Levitt, 1976); 2) teachers are quite reactive to the demands and added burdens imposed by handicapped children who are difficult to teach and manage (Lynn, 1981); and 3) the attitudes of regular teachers toward mainstreaming are consistently less positive than those of special educators and nonteaching personnel such as school psychologists and special education directors. Further, research by Dwiggins (1981) indicates that teachers do not adjust their behavioral standards downward to accommodate mildly and severely handicapped children. This suggests the possibility that handicapped children are all too often mainstreamed into the classrooms of teachers whose behavioral standards they could not possibly meet.

Keogh and Levitt (1976) report that regular teachers are also quite concerned about 1) having control over who is mainstreamed into their classrooms; 2) their ability to meet the needs of mainstreamed handicapped children; and 3) the availability of support services and technical assistance. These concerns are not surprising. In fact, they are to be expected, given the relative isolation of regular teachers from the broad range of handicapped children.

Of equal or, perhaps, greater significance to the development of handicapped children, is their ability to cope with the pressures and demands of the peer groups they encounter within mainstream settings. One of the major assumptions underlying P.L. 94-142 was that through exposure to nonhandicapped peers, mainstreamed handicapped children would 1) be exposed to normal standards and patterns of behavior; 2) acquire social skills and improve their social competence; and 3) engage in social participation with nonhandicapped peers. What is the research evidence on these questions?

It appears that as a field we have greatly underestimated the complexities involved in developing social and academic competence among populations of integrated handicapped children. The extent to which such children would be socially rejected by peers, excluded from social participation, and negatively reacted to by receiving teachers was totally unexpected by the framers and advocates of P.L. 94-142 (Allen, Benning, & Drummond, 1972; Larrivee & Cook, 1979). Convergent evidence across a large number of studies (see Gresham, 1981; Guralnick, 1981) indicates that handicapped children interact with nonhandicapped children at extremely low rates in mainstream settings, and that a large percentage of the social interactions that do occur are negative in nature! Evidence also suggests that the more severe the handicapping condition, the lower the rate of social contact, interaction, and participation with peers.

In addition, studies of the mainstreaming process indicate that handicapped children are *not* accepted by their nonhandicapped peers. These findings have been demonstrated across both varying types (Learning Disabled, Educable Mentally Retarded, Emotionally Disabled) and severity levels of handicapping conditions (Bryan & Wheeler, 1972; Iano, Ayers, Heller, McGettigan, & Walker, 1974). And finally, there is evidence that nonintegrated handicapped children are better accepted by their nonhandicapped peers than are mainstreamed handicapped children (Gottlieb & Budoff, 1973) and that the more time handicapped children spend in less restrictive settings, the more likely they are to be socially rejected by peers (Gottlieb, 1978).

To date, integration has been considered largely successful if the handicapped child is involved in interactive exchanges with nonhandicapped peers in normalized social environments, and participates (at whatever level of involvement the teacher can accommodate) in classroom activities. It is clear from the evidence accumulated in the last decade that this is a most inappropriate standard for judging the success of mainstreaming efforts. Further, Gresham (1982) reviews evidence that suggests that mainstreamed handicapped children *do not* naturally model the behavior of their nonhandicapped peers. Thus, mere placement of the handicapped child in a less restrictive setting will probably not lead to normalized behavior and improved social competence (Peck, Cooke, & Apolloni, 1981). This is one of the major assumptions upon which P.L. 94-142 was based, and one that appears, in retrospect, to be unsupportable by available evidence.

There is considerable research indicating that the self-esteem and academic achievement of mainstreamed handicapped children are not superior to that of nonintegrated children (Budoff & Gottlieb, 1976). Moreover, the evidence is overwhelming as to their lack of social acceptance by, and social participation with, nonhandicapped peers. If we consider *both* the quality of educational program and restrictiveness of setting features of the LRE provision (Lowenbraun & Affleck, 1979), then it is clear that we have not, and currently are not, succeeding in our efforts. In too many cases mainstreaming turns out to be a stressful, negative, and often unpleasant experience for the handicapped child, receiving teacher, nonhandicapped peers, and especially for the child's parents.

These outcomes are no doubt due, in part, to the lack of experience of nonhandicapped peers and regular teachers in accommodating handicapped children. For example, Forness (S. Forness, personal communication, 1982) provides evidence suggesting that teachers' evaluations of, and responses to, mainstreamed handicapped children can act as mediating variables that negatively influence peers' evaluations of the handicapped child's social and academic competence. However, the available evidence strongly suggests that such outcomes are also influenced by the actual behavior that handicapped children display in mainstream settings (Bruininks, 1978; MacMillan & Morrison, 1980). For example, deaf preschoolers rely much more on physical contact, approval, and negative interaction than normal students (Van Lieshout, 1973). Learning disabled students, compared to normals, are less able to present convincing arguments to their peers (Bryan, Donahue, & Pearl, 1980), have fewer interactions with them (Bryan, 1974), and exhibit more aggressive/negative behaviors than their peers (Bryan & Bryan, 1978). Handicapped children are also perceived by their peers as being less academically competent and intellectually capable, deficient in communicative/verbal skills, and as exhibiting higher levels of antisocial behavior and aggression than their nonhandicapped peers (Gottlieb, 1978).

Collectively, these findings suggest that the mainstreaming process is not resulting in the positive outcomes that were anticipated for either handicapped children or their nonhandicapped peers. In fact, the exact opposite appears to be true. Many artifacts of the mainstreaming process include unexpected negative outcomes. Often, mainstreaming seems to result in the handicapped child being placed in a more, rather than less, restrictive social environment (Gresham, 1981).

Traditional Approaches to LRE Placements in School Settings

The literature on the handicapped child, LRE, and the mainstreaming-integration process is replete with discussions of strategies for involving handicapped children in social interactive-participatory processes with nonhandicapped children in the least restrictive setting possible (Guralnick, 1978). Allen (1981) described curriculum models and presented teaching guidelines for achieving this goal within mainstreaming, reverse mainstreaming, and transitional school classroom settings. Research has demonstrated the efficacy of several approaches for involving preschool and school age handicapped children in social interactions with nonhandicapped peers, including *behavioral* (Allen et al., 1972), *ecological* (Rogers-Warren & Warren, 1977), and *Piagetian* (Bricker & Bricker, 1976) models.

There is little question or argument regarding the importance of peer interactions and social contacts to the socialization process. Hartup (1979), for example, has eloquently described the contributions of peer-to-peer social interactions to the development of social competence in *normal* children. He argues that without an opportunity to interact with peers, children have difficulty in learning effective communication skills, modulating aggressive feelings, accommodating to social demands for appropriate sexual behavior, and forming a coherent set of moral values. It appears that adults and same-age peers make unique contributions to the socialization process with prosocial and cooperative behavioral competencies derived primarily from peer interactions.

It is the authors' contention that the simple exposure of socially unskilled handicapped children to interactive opportunities with nonhandicapped peer groups may be a necessary, but insufficient condition for the development of social competence, and the simple integration of handicapped children into regular academic settings will not automatically produce improved academic competence. As noted above, studies of the mainstreaming process across a broad range of handicapping conditions, settings, and age ranges indicate that natural contingencies controlled by nonhandicapped peers and teachers in less restrictive settings do not, in the majority of cases, produce identifiable benefits for handicapped children placed within them (Gottlieb, 1978;

Gresham, 1981, 1982). It is essential that school-age handicapped children be directly taught the skills that determine social and behavioral competence, and that support systems be developed to facilitate the development of these skills into more complex behavioral repertoires over time.

Necessary Conditions Governing Effective Social Integration Into LRE School Settings

As the literature on the deleterious effects of mainstreaming has become available and known to parents and professionals, there have been numerous calls for the systematic training of mainstreamed handicapped children in social skills that will improve social competence and lead to peer acceptance. Guralnick (1978) argues that improved social skills should lead to greater interactive opportunities and, possibly, greater social acceptance from nonhandicapped peers. This may be more likely for the mildly handicapped (Ladd, 1981). For example, Fredericks, Baldwin, Grove, Moore, Riggs, and Lyons (1978), in reporting a model program for the integration of preschool severely handicapped children into mainstream settings, commented extensively on the complexity of this process, and the degree of staff training, resource support, and direct assistance and supervision required to ensure a successful mainstreaming effort.

The authors contend that for mainstreaming to be successful across a variety of settings and handicapped populations, including preschool handicapped children, we must be willing to invest in a much greater and more systematic preparation of the child and receiving setting. At an absolute minimum, in the mainstreaming process and in the preparation of handicapped children for entry into regular settings, we need to attend carefully to the four sets of influences identified by Gottlieb (1978) that can shape the quality of children's successful social adaptation in school. These are: 1) the child's observable behavior; 2) characteristics of the peer group; 3) the observable reactions of the teacher who establishes and enforces norms of appropriate behavior for the class; and 4) the environmental setting. In other words, a workable solution to this overall problem involves far more than the direct training of a young handicapped child in an array of social skills via a social skills curriculum that is presumed to influence social competence. To accomplish this important objective, a methodology is needed that will

1) identify functional social skills predictive of social competence;

2) develop measures to identify socially incompetent children and assess their status and deficits underlying their incompetence;
3) construct a social skills curriculum that can be used effectively by teachers and parents;
4) provide opportunities for demonstration and further development of target social skills in natural settings;
5) motivate peers to support the child's attempts at using these skills; and
6) incorporate features to ensure the durability and generalizability (over time and settings) of improved social competence and behavior changes.

A methodology incorporating all these elements does not currently exist.

The social skills literature contains a few examples of controlled experiments wherein cognitive and social skills training procedures have improved the social acceptance of nonhandicapped (Gottman, Gonso, & Schuler, 1976) and mildly handicapped children (Gresham, 1981). However, studies showing a measurable impact on the observable behavior of such children are extremely rare (O'Connor, 1969), and often do not replicate when they are obtained (Gottman, 1977). The question of the long-term impact of social skills training on social acceptance remains to be demonstrated with both normal and mildly handicapped children (Hops, in press).

At present we do not know the level and amount of training necessary to impact the social behavior repertoires and corresponding acceptance of handicapped children. However, at a minimum, it is likely to require both cognitive and behavioral mastery of specific social skills with opportunities for the skills to be demonstrated and directly reinforced within natural settings (Hops, in press). Walker, McConnell, Walker et al. (1983) and McConnell (1982) found that behavior management procedures were essential to ensure mastery and actual use of cognitively taught social skills. In addition, it was necessary to restructure and program the child's social environment to support the handicapped child's attempts at applying the skills.

Walker and his colleagues (Hersh & Walker, 1983; Walker, McConnell, Walker et al., 1983; Walker & Rankin, 1983) are currently refining a systematic approach to mainstreaming children in the elementary grades that incorporates social systems and ecological perspectives and directly addresses two of the four sets of influences identified by Gottlieb (1979); i.e., the observable behavior of the handicapped child to be mainstreamed, and the observable reactions of the receiving teacher(s) who establishes and enforces norms of appropriate behavior.

A service delivery model has been developed for the mainstreaming process, focusing on the social behavior of handicapped children, that contains the following components: an ecological assessment system, a social skills curriculum, and a behavior management system. The conceptual rationale for this approach to the mainstreaming process grows out of several literatures, including those on

1) teacher expectations and their behavioral expression (Brophy & Evertson, 1981);
2) classroom ecology (Copeland, 1980);
3) generalization of behavior changes across time and setting (O'Leary & O'Leary, 1976);
4) problems associated with the mainstreaming process (Gresham, 1981); and
5) the authors' direct experience with the mainstreaming-reintegration process over a nine-year period (Hops, Walker, & Greenwood, 1979).

This methodology can be used as a guide both in selecting appropriate less restrictive school settings and in preparing handicapped children for the behavioral demands and expectations that exist within these settings.

THE SBS MODEL PROGRAM: A SYSTEMATIC APPROACH TO THE
INTEGRATION OF HANDICAPPED CHILDREN INTO LESS RESTRICTIVE
SETTINGS

The SBS Model Program focuses on the *placement* and *integration* components of P.L. 94-142. It provides a methodology for the social integration of handicapped children into less restrictive settings, and seeks to improve the child's adjustment capability in classroom and freeplay settings. Specifically, the program's major goals are:

1) To select appropriate placement settings for the integration of mildly and moderately handicapped children into the educational mainstream.
2) To identify the minimal behavioral skills and competencies required

for a successful classroom adjustment in the target settings, and to identify the noxious social behaviors that are unacceptable to teachers.

3) To prepare such children to meet the receiving teacher's behavioral expectations and to achieve adjustment to nonhandicapped peer groups.

As noted above, the results of mainstreaming research indicate that handicapped children often experience significant difficulty in adjusting to the behavioral demands of regular teachers in less restrictive settings and in developing peer-to-peer social relationships that lead to social interaction with and acceptance by nonhandicapped peers. Further, teachers in mainstream settings have expressed grave reservations concerning their ability to meet the needs of mainstreamed handicapped children and the availability of support services and technical assistance to facilitate the process. The SBS Program was designed to address these problems.

The major thrust of mainstreaming efforts to date has been to encourage the receiving target setting to accommodate to the handicapped child's skill deficits and needs. This process places a great deal of pressure on the management and instructional skills of teachers in mainstream settings, and has achieved only limited success in exposing handicapped children to the potential benefits of social integration. The SBS Program distributes the demands and logistical burdens of the mainstreaming process more evenly between the *sending* (special education) setting and the *receiving* (regular education) setting by 1) assessing the behavioral demands and expectations of less restrictive settings; 2) using this information to select potential mainstream placement settings and to prepare the target child to meet the demands/expectations prior to actual integrations; 3) identifying the receiving teacher's technical assistance needs in teaching and managing the handicapped child following integration; and 4) providing resource support and technical assistance services to ensure a continuing successful mainstreaming experience for the handicapped child, receiving teacher(s), and peers (Walker, 1984).

SBS Program Components

The SBS Program has two major components: assessment and intervention. They can be used separately or in combination. When used together, they make it possible to assess the behavioral demands and expectations of less restrictive settings, assess the target child's behavioral status in relation to those standards, and prepare the handicapped child to cope with these standards prior to actual integration.

Assessment. The SBS assessment component, AIMS (**A**ssessment for **I**ntegration into **M**ainstream **S**ettings) is designed for use in:

1) the selection of mainstream settings;
2) identifying the adaptive skills and competencies required in the receiving setting, and the noxious social behaviors judged to be unacceptable by the receiving teacher; and
3) generating information on the receiving teachers' technical assistance needs in teaching and managing the mainstreamed child.

The AIMS system contains four instruments. These are: *The SBS Inventory of Teacher Social Behavior Standards and Expectations, The SBS Checklist of Correlates of Child Handicapping Conditions, The Social Interaction Code (SIC),* and *The Classroom Adjustment Code (CAC).* The first two instruments are used to provide an ecological assessment of potential mainstream settings prior to integration. The latter two are used to provide direct assessments of the adequacy of the target child's behavioral adjustment in classroom and freeplay settings following integration.

In the *SBS Inventory* teachers are asked to evaluate dimensions of adaptive and maladaptive child behavior, and to indicate their technical assistance needs in teaching/managing children who are deficient in adaptive skills and competencies and outside the normal range on maladaptive social behaviors. Teachers rate descriptions of adaptive child behaviors (e.g., makes his or her assistance needs known in an appropriate manner) in terms of whether they are critical, desirable, or unimportant to a successful classroom adjustment. Similarly, item descriptions of maladaptive behavior (e.g., child refuses to obey teacher-imposed classroom rules) are rated as unacceptable, tolerated, or acceptable. The resulting information can be used in the selection of placement settings and as a tool in teaching required mainstream behavioral competencies.

The *SBS Correlates Checklist* identifies conditions and characteristics often associated with disabilities that could cause teachers to resist placement of handicapped children who manifest them. *The Classroom Adjustment (CAC)* and *Social Interaction (SIC)* observation codes are both interval recording systems and are designed for use in assessing the handicapped child's classroom and peer-to-peer adjustment status following integration. The SIC provides information on three major variables; i.e., a measure of structure, and categories of both appropriate and inappropriate interactive behavior in freeplay settings. The SIC yields measures on the quality of interactive behavior, the amount of social participation, and the degree of verbal content in social exchanges. The CAC provides information on three categories of child behavior and five categories of teacher behavior. These codes make it possible to measure the child's classroom adjustment status and to determine the type and amount of teacher behavior directed toward the child.

Approximately four years have been invested in the development, revision, refinement, and validation of these instruments. Ten studies have been completed on the SBS Inventory and Checklist, and an equal number are in progress. The SBS instrument development process and initial validation studies are described in Walker and Rankin (1983). The SIC and CAC are completed and their reliability established. They will be published in a forthcoming report.

Intervention. A social skills training program called ACCEPTS (**A** Curriculum for Children's Effective Peer and Teacher Skills) (Walker, McConnell, Holmes et al., 1983) was developed to teach social skills judged essential for coping with the adjustment demands of mainstream settings. The ACCEPTS Program can be used either independently or in collaboration with the AIMS assessment system, and contains the following elements: 1) a nine-step instructional procedure based on principles of direct instruction; 2) scripts for teaching four critically important teacher-child behavioral competencies and 24 peer-to-peer social skills; 3) videotaped examples of skills being taught and applied and non-examples of the skills being incorrectly applied; 4) behavior management procedures for use during the teaching process and for strengthening correct application of the skills in playground and classroom settings; and 5) guidelines for using the curriculum and for training others to implement it. The program teaches social skills and uses coaching and behavior management procedures to facilitate demonstration of the target skills in natural settings.

The ACCEPTS curriculum teaches two major types of social skills: 1) critical classroom behaviors that contribute to a successful classroom adjustment as defined by teachers; e.g., listening to instructions, following directions, making assistance needs known in an appropriate manner; and 2) peer-to-peer social skills that contribute to social competence and peer acceptance; e.g., basic interaction skills, conversation skills, knowledge of how to make friends, and so forth. Social skills are defined by the authors as social responses that allow one to initiate and maintain positive relationships with others, contribute to peer acceptance and to a successful classroom adjustment, and allow one to cope effectively and adaptively with the social environment.

Table 1 lists the skills taught by the ACCEPTS curriculum. The authors devoted considerable time, effort, and research attention to

TABLE 1
ACCEPTS Social Skills

AREA I. CLASSROOM SKILLS
    1) Listening to the Teacher
    2) When the Teacher Asks You to Do Something
    3) Doing Your Best Work
    4) Following the Classroom Rules

AREA II. BASIC INTERACTION SKILLS
    1) Eye Contact
    2) Using the Right Voice
    3) Starting
    4) Listening
    5) Answering
    6) Making Sense
    7) Taking Turns Talking
    8) A Question
    9) Continuing

AREA III. GETTING ALONG SKILLS
    1) Using Polite Words
    2) Sharing
    3) Following Rules
    4) Assisting Others
    5) Touching the Right Way

AREA IV. MAKING FRIENDS SKILLS
    1) Good Grooming
    2) Smiling
    3) Complimenting
    4) Friendship Making

AREA V. COPING SKILLS
    1) When Someone Says "No"
    2) When You Express Anger
    3) When Someone Teases You
    4) When Someone Tries to Hurt You
    5) When Someone Asks You to Do Something You Can't Do
    6) When Things Don't Go Right

---

selection of the *classroom* and *peer-to-peer* skills included in the AC-CEPTS curriculum. As part of the SBS Program's larger focus, over 1,500 teachers in the U.S. and Canada responded to a rating instrument that required them to rate the importance of 56 adaptive behaviors in facilitating a successful classroom adjustment. There was broad consensus within and among the teacher groups making up the sample as to the most and least important behavioral competencies. The most consistently high-rated items across teachers were incorporated into the ACCEPTS curriculum under the Classroom Skills content area.

The peer-to-peer social skills were selected using three methods: a review of the existing literature on the identification of key social skills discriminating between socially competent and incompetent children (e.g., Gottman et al., 1975), a review and analysis of the social skills taught and outcomes achieved within social skills training programs reported in the literature (e.g., LaGreca & Santogrossi, 1980), and a logical analysis of the skills and competencies that would be required for handicapped children to cope effectively with the social demands of mainstream settings. The list of social skills also incorporates those behavioral areas and specific skills that have been empirically related to social competence as measured by sociometric tests (Gottman et al., 1975). In the social skills area, these include: knowledge of how to make friends, communication skills, and distributing and receiving positive social behavior.

Curricula material and instructional procedures are incorporated into the ACCEPTS curriculum for all of these skills. Attempts were made to select an array of skills that would be functional, relevant, teachable, and of sufficient breadth to influence social-behavioral competence.

EFFICACY AND VALIDATION STUDIES OF THE ACCEPTS SOCIAL SKILLS TRAINING PROGRAM

Three experiments are reported herein relating to the development, testing, revision, and validation of the ACCEPTS social skills program. Studies One and Two are experimental. Study Three is descriptive in nature.

Study One: Initial Evaluation of the ACCEPTS Program

The original prototype version of the ACCEPTS Program was investigated in this study (Walker, McConnell, Holmes et al., 1983).

Twenty-eight mildly/moderately handicapped children participated in an experimental study of the program's effects over a two- to three-month period. The study sample was recruited from the elementary handicapped population of the Eugene, Oregon school district. Teachers and psychologists referred 34 students judged to be in need of social skills training. All were certified as handicapped. Twenty-seven of the referred subjects completed the study and were included in the data analysis.

The handicapping conditions of learning disabled (15), educable mentally retarded (1), language impaired (7), emotionally handicapped (1), multiply handicapped (1), and neurologically impaired (3) were included in the study sample. All but three of the subjects were enrolled in special or resource room settings as their primary classroom placement.

A post-only control group design was used to investigate effects of the independent variable in this study (Campbell & Stanley, 1963). Referred handicapped children were randomly assigned to either a control group or one of two experimental groups.

Children in Experimental Group One were exposed to the social skills training program accompanied by contingency management procedures applied within playground and classroom settings. Experimental Group Two subjects were exposed to the social skills training program only. Control subjects received no social skills or contingency management training during this study.

A standardized procedure was used to teach the four classroom and 24 peer-to-peer social skills to children in the two experimental groups. The instructional procedure included the following elements: 1) a verbal definition of the skill, illustrative examples, and discussion of its use; 2) symbolic modeling of instances and non-instances of the skill by videotaped, same-age peer models; 3) practice of the skills in role play situations and activities with feedback, correction, and social praise supplied by the instructor; and 4) presentation of a criterion role play situation to assess whether the target child had mastered the skill at an acceptable level. Approximately 45 minutes per day were devoted to instruction in the ACCEPTS Program.

A contingency management program was added to the instructional procedures for subjects assigned to Experimental Group One. This component was designed to provide coaching and reinforcement of the previously taught skills within natural interactive settings such as the playground and classroom. The 10 subjects within Experimental Group One received complete instruction in the ACCEPTS curriculum, as well as reinforcement (social praise and freetime activity rewards) for displaying newly acquired skills in natural settings. The contingency was individually applied to the behavior of the 10 subjects in Experimental Group One. Earned freetime rewards were also provided on an individual basis.

Instructors of target handicapped children in this study included three project staff members and six graduate students in special education or school psychology. These individuals each taught social skills to two or three of the children, and applied contingency management procedures to their playground and classroom behavior if assigned to Experimental Group One. Each trainer completed the entire curriculum with the same group of two or three children who were taught in separate small group sessions.

Four steps were taken to maximize the consistency of implementation across the nine trainers. First, all trainers were familiarized with the purpose and rationale of the model program and the study. Second, trainers thoroughly reviewed the ACCEPTS curriculum, training materials, and videotapes. Third, trainers were instructed in the use of the standardized instructional procedure described by project staff members. Each trainer practiced applying this instructional procedure in role play situations, and corrective feedback was provided on their performance. Finally, frequent meetings and consultations were held during the training phase of the study to answer questions, provide feedback, and monitor progress of the trainers.

Two of the trainers served as resource persons and coordinators of the implementation process. Considerable amounts of informal monitoring and training were provided to other trainers by these individuals.

Three major dependent variables were recorded in this study: teacher ratings, a behavioral role play test, and behavioral observation data recorded in natural settings. Subjects' *classroom* behavior was assessed via teacher ratings and direct behavioral observations recorded in the classroom. The subjects' peer-oriented *social* behavior was assessed via teacher ratings, a behavioral role play test, and direct observations recorded in playground settings. All these measures were administered at post-only; i.e., after all treatment procedures were terminated.

Reliabilities on the observational code categories contained in the *Classroom* and *Social Interaction Codes* were consistently in the .80–.90 range. Reliability information was not available for teacher ratings and the behavioral role play test.

Results favored the two experimental groups over the control group on all three dependent measures. However, statistically significant differences were obtained only on the criterion role play test and classroom observation data. The percent of role play skills correctly displayed by Group One, Two, and Control subjects were, respectively, 72.8%, 70.43%, and 58% ($p < .009$). Similarly, on the classroom observations measure, both Group One and Two subjects averaged 80% of observed intervals on-task, while control subjects averaged 62% ($p < .04$).

One of three interactive measures (interactive inappropriate) derived from playground observations approached significance at $p < .06$. No significant differences were obtained between the two experimental groups on any of the three classes of dependent measures. However, Group One children were favored on teacher ratings of classroom and peer-to-peer skills, as well as playground observations.

These initial evaluation results were encouraging, but also suggested areas in which the intervention procedures could be strengthened. The intervention package was revised to improve its teachability, power, and instructional precision. The revision included a more powerful curriculum and the addition of group contingencies to the behavior management system to involve peers more directly in the process of improving the social-behavioral competence of target handicapped children.

Study Two: Replication and Further Evaluation of ACCEPTS

Study Two evaluated the effects of the revised and expanded version of the ACCEPTS Program. A pre-post experimental control group design was used for this purpose.

Twenty handicapped children enrolled in grades two through five participated in Study Two. All were enrolled in regular classroom settings and were certified as handicapped. Both severity levels and types of handicapping conditions were approximately equivalent in the samples for Studies One and Two. The 20 subjects were randomly assigned to either the experimental or the control group.

Experimental group children were instructed in the revised ACCEPTS Program in the same way Study One children were. Experimental group subjects received 1) daily instruction in the ACCEPTS Program social skills; 2) individual contingency management procedures to increase the use of classroom skills; and 3) coaching and group contingency management procedures to increase social participation and to support use of the previously taught social skills. Control subjects received no training in social skills. Instructional procedures were identical from Study One to Two.

Measures were also identical in Studies One and Two. Teacher ratings and behavioral observations of peer-to-peer social skills in free play settings were collected for all children at four time points: before training, during training, immediately following the end of training, and at two-month follow-up. Classroom observations were recorded before, during, and immediately following training. A criterion role play test was completed by all participating children (experimental and control) immediately after training.

As in Study One, the results showed significantly higher performance levels for experimental subjects on the criterion role play test. Teacher ratings from pre to post showed essentially no change for experimental subjects, and a slight increase for control subjects. Statistically significant changes were achieved for experimental subjects on three measures derived from direct observations of their behavior in classroom and playground settings: percent of time on-task (classroom), percent of time spent engaged in social participation with peers (playground), and percent of total interactive behavior having verbal content. Statistically significant Group by Time interactions were obtained for each of these direct observation measures.

Table 2 presents means, standard deviations, and ranges for experimental and control subjects on the dependent measures used in the study. Table 3 summarizes results of the analyses for each variable.

There were dramatic increases from *pre* to *during* for experimental subjects on all three direct observation measures (see Table 2). For the on-task variable, the levels at *during* and *post* were approximately identical. For percent social, there was a loss of six percentage points from *during* to *post*. There was an even more dramatic loss of 16 percentage points from *during* to *post* on the percent verbal measure.

At follow-up, the percent social level had further dropped to just below its *pre* level (79% versus 81%). There was a four percentage point gain from *post* to *follow-up* for the percent verbal measure (26% to 30%).

Control subjects' levels on the percent verbal measure were relatively stable across the four time points. However, on both the percent social and on-task measures, there was a gradual increase across the four time points. Despite random assignment, the control subjects' means were considerably higher on the percent social and verbal measures at *pre*.

The authors have no explanation for the dramatic drop-off for ex-

TABLE 2
Means and Ranges of the Dependent Measures in Study Two

		PRE			DURING			POST			FOLLOWUP	
		M	S.D.	Range	M	S.D.	Range	M	S.D.	Range	M	S.D.	Range
Percent Skills, Role Play Test	Treatment							.842	.070	.73-.96			
	Control							.379	.303	.04-.65			
Classroom Skills, Teacher Rating	Treatment	11.11	3.14	7-17				11.56	4.00	7-17	11.13	5.52	5-20
	Control	9.00	2.39	7-14				9.80	2.62	4-13	9.78	2.86	5-13
Peer Skills, Teacher Rating	Treatment	60.44	7.02	47-69				65.78	12.04	46-88	59.63	12.86	33-74
	Control	57.38	15.53	32-85				55.30	17.49	29-82	60.00	13.68	35-86
Percent On-Task, Direct Observation	Treatment	.681	.149	.42-.88	.859	.116	.64-.98	.848	.100	.67-.97			
	Control	.698	.124	.48-.84	.717	.119	.52-.90	.770	.078	.64-.89			
Percent Social, Direct Observation	Treatment	.816	.244	.29-.99	.987	.023	.94-1.00	.925	.071	.77-1.00	.792	.303	.00-1.00
	Control	.868	.079	.68-.94	.876	.111	.66-.99	.915	.087	.71-1.00	.934	.084	.74-1.00
Percent Verbal, Direct Observation	Treatment	.229	.149	.06-.56	.409	.148	.21-.69	.260	.093	.09-.41	.300	.184	.00-.69
	Control	.330	.110	.17-.49	.296	.113	.09-.43	.359	.170	.12-.58	.362	.151	.04-.55

TABLE 3

Summary of Repeated Measures Analyses of Variance in Study Two

Measure	Group	Time	Group × Time
Classroom Skills, Teacher Rating[1]	1.93 $p = .191$	.12 $p = .89$	.05 $p = .952$
Peer Skills, Teacher Rating[1]	.02 $p = .890$	.55[2] $p = .583$	.26 $p = .777$
Percent on Task, Direct Observation[2]	3.38 $p = .083$	8.06 $p = .001$	3.13 $p = .056$
Percent Social, Direct Observation[2]	.20 $p = .659$	1.80 $p = .157$	2.72 $p = .053$
Percent Verbal, Direct Observation[2]	.78 $p = .389$	1.28 $p = .292$	3.36 $p = .025$

[1]Degrees of Freedom: Group (1, 12), Time (2, 24), Group × Time (2, 24).
[2]Degrees of Freedom: Group (1, 18), Time (3, 54), Group × Time (3, 54).

perimental subjects from *during* to *post* on the percent verbal measure, and from *post* to *follow-up* on the percent social measure. Careful studies of the factors accounting for such outcomes and of maintenance/generalization procedures for remediating them are clearly needed.

These findings are in stark contrast to those reported by Oden and Asher (1977), who investigated the use of coaching in teaching social skills to nonhandicapped children. Coaching was instrumental in increasing target subjects' peer acceptance, and those gains were maintained at a one-year follow-up. Coaching procedures were used in both Studies One and Two reported here, but did not produce maintenance of achieved gains. It is possible that maintenance and generalization processes are far more complex with handicapped than nonhandicapped populations.

An individual analysis of the data for the experimental group subjects revealed that there was a clear maintenance effect for five of the 10 subjects. Maintenance was greatest for those subjects who had the lowest initial levels on the three direct observation measures; e.g., below 50%.

A final factor that could have affected the maintenance levels achieved concerns a relative lack of support by the regular teachers for the social skills training procedure. The majority of teachers in whose classes the target experimental subjects were enrolled saw the social skills training procedures as intruding on the existing academic program. Furthermore, they assigned a low priority to the social skills training of mainstreamed handicapped children, as indicated by verbal comments made to the program's trainers. It is possible that this relative lack of teacher support could have contributed to the failure to achieve maintenance effects.

Study Three: Development of a Normative Data Base and Social Validation of ACCEPTS Behavioral Gains

This study focused on developing a normative data base on the SIC and CAC observation codes described earlier for use in socially validating social skills gains and generating a standard for evaluating the adequacy of handicapped children's adjustment status in mainstream settings (Kazdin, 1977; Walker & Hops, 1976). These data make it possible to socially validate the results of Studies One and Two.

The subjects for Study Three were 12 elementary-aged pupils in grades one through six. The children ranged in age from six to 11 years; seven were males and five were females. All were enrolled in mainstream regular classrooms. Twelve teachers were asked to nominate three pupils from their classes who were of a normal social skill level and of average social status. One out of each group of three nominated students was randomly selected to participate in the study. The 12 children were observed in both playground and classroom settings. On the playground, observations were recorded during morning or noon recesses within ongoing freeplay activities. In classroom settings, the same subjects were observed during seatwork periods.

Children were observed for a minimum of three one-hour sessions in both playground and classroom settings scheduled on separate days. They were observed on the SIC in playground settings and on the CAC in classroom settings. These codes were also used in Studies One and Two as one of three dependent measures.

Five reliability sessions were conducted during the study. All produced mean agreement ratios in the .80-.90 range on both codes. Table 4 contains means and ranges for the 12 children on four variables derived from the observation data. Observation sessions were combined

TABLE 4

Means and Ranges for the Direct Observation Measures in Study Three

	M	S.D.	Range
Percent Social	.984	.020	.94-1.00
Percent Verbal	.479	.125	.23- .64
Percent Inappropriate Social Behavior	.002	.004	.00- .01
Percent On Task	.903	—*	.63- .99

Note: $n = 12$
*Data not available

for each subject, and then averaged across subjects to obtain these figures. The results indicate that children in this sample were socially participating almost continuously in freeplay settings, engaged in verbal content during approximately half of their social exchanges, had an extremely low rate of inappropriate social behavior, and engaged in appropriate on-task classroom behavior approximately 90% of the time.

Table 5 presents comparative data (post) on these four variables for the two experimental subject groups in Study One, and for experimental subjects across the four time points of Study Two.

The data in Table 5 indicate that subjects in Study One were well below normative levels at the post time point. The comparative data for Study Two experimental subjects suggest that the revised version of the ACCEPTS Program was more powerful than the initial version. A very powerful *during* effect was achieved for all four variables in Study Two that approximated normative levels. However, as already noted, these levels were not maintained.

The normative data reported in this study are valuable for the purposes cited above; i.e., social validation of treatment gains and evaluation of adjustment status. However, the generalizability and representativeness of these data are constrained by the small sample size ($n = 12$). Replication of these results with larger samples is clearly indicated.

TABLE 5
Experimental Subjects' Comparative Performance on Selected
Outcome Variables With a Normative Standard

Variable	Percent Social	Percent Verbal	Inappropriate Social Behavior	Percent On Task
Normative Level	.984	.479	.002	.903
Study One Experimental Group One	.825	.290	.011	.807
Experimental Group Two	.810	.337	.052	.803
Study Two Experimental Group Pre	.816	.229	.018	.681
During	.987	.409	.003	.859
Post	.925	.260	.007	.848
Follow-up	.792	.300	—*	—*

*Data not available

GENERAL DISCUSSION

The studies reported herein demonstrate that a combination of cognitively taught social skills and contingency management procedures applied in natural settings can be used to improve the classroom and social adjustments of handicapped children. These outcomes were demonstrated in both self-contained (Study One) and regular (Study Two) classroom and playground settings. However, the effects of exposure to the ACCEPTS Program on peer acceptance were not assessed in this study. In the authors' view, social skills training programs must ultimately be tested against this standard if they are to be properly evaluated.

The normative comparisons in Study Three suggest that powerful programs such as ACCEPTS must be applied over a substantial length of time to move handicapped children to within the normal range. Maintaining these gains over the longer term and facilitating their transfer to non-intervention settings represent complex problems that warrant systematic investigation. In this context, Gresham (1981) notes that training for generalization should receive as much attention as training for the acquisition of social skills if mainstreaming efforts are to be successful.

Study Two is one of the few reported investigations to date of social skills training with handicapped children enrolled in mainstream settings. The authors' experience suggests that powerful logistical barriers may impinge upon this process. How they are negotiated will determine the ultimate feasibility of conducting systematic social skills training in mainstream settings.

SUMMARY

The results of the literature reviewed and studies reported herein suggest that 1) handicapped children experience significant adjustment problems upon entry into mainstream settings, 2) systematic procedures are usually not implemented to prevent and ameliorate such problems, and 3) a substantial investment of time, effort and expertise is required to ensure that the social integration process is a positive one for mainstreamed handicapped children. Very few investigators have been able to demonstrate enduring changes in the sociometric status and social adjustment of handicapped children enrolled in less restrictive educational settings.

REFERENCES

ALEXANDER, C., & STRAIN, P. (1978). A review of educators' attitudes toward handicapped children and the concept of mainstreaming. *Psychology in the Schools, 15*, 390-396.

ALLEN, K. E. (1981). Curriculum models for successful mainstreaming. *Topics in Early Childhood Education, 1*, 45-56.

ALLEN, K. E., BENNING, P. M., & DRUMMOND, T. W. (1972). Integration of normal and handicapped children in a behavior modification preschool: A case study. In G. Semb (Ed.), *Behavior analysis and education*. Lawrence, KS: University of Kansas Press.

ASHER, S. R., & GOTTMAN, J. M. (Eds.). (1981). *The development of children's friendships*. Cambridge: Cambridge University Press.

ASHER, S. R., & TAYLOR, A. (1981). Social outcomes of mainstreaming: Sociometric assessment and beyond. *Aspen Systems Corporation*, 13-30.

BLOOM, B. S. (1976). *Human characteristics and school learning*. New York: McGraw-Hill.

BRICKER, W., & BRICKER, D. (1976). The infant, toddler, and preschool research and intervention project. In T. Tjossem (Ed.), *Intervention strategies with at-risk infants and young children.* Baltimore: University Park Press.

BRONSON, W. C. (1966). Central orientations: A study of behavior organization from childhood to adolescence. *Child Development, 37,* 125-255.

BROPHY, J. E., & EVERTSON, C. (1981). *Student characteristics and teaching.* New York: Longman.

BROPHY, J. E., & GOOD, T. (1970). Teachers' communication of differential expectations for children's classroom performance: Some behavioral data. *Journal of Educational Psychology, 61,* 365-374.

BRUININKS, V. L. (1978). Peer status and personality characteristics of learning disabled and nondisabled students. *Journal of Learning Disabilities, 11,* 484-489.

BRYAN, T. S. (1974). Peer popularity of learning disabled children. *Journal of Learning Disabilities, 7,* 621-625.

BRYAN, T., & BRYAN, J. (1978). Social interactions of learning disabled children. *Learning Disability Quarterly, 1,* 33-38.

BRYAN, T., DONAHUE, M., & PEARL, R. (1980, May). *Learning disabled children's peer interactions during a small group problem-solving task.* Paper presented at the meeting of the Association for Behavior Analysis, Dearborn, Michigan.

BRYAN, T. S., & WHEELER, R. (1972). Perception of children with learning disabilities: The eye of the observer. *Journal of Learning Disabilities, 5,* 484-488.

BUDOFF, M., & GOTTLIEB, J. (1976). Special class EMR children mainstreamed: A study of an aptitude (learning potential) × treatment interaction. *American Journal of Mental Deficiency, 81,* 1-11.

CAMPBELL, D., & STANLEY, J. (1963). *Experimental and quasi-experimental designs for research.* Chicago: Rand McNally.

COBB, J. A., & HOPS, H. (1973). Effects of academic survival skills training on low achieving first graders. *Journal of Educational Research, 67,* 108-113.

COPELAND, W. D. (1980). Teaching-learning behaviors and the demands of the classroom environment. *The Elementary School Journal, 80,* 163-177.

COWEN, E., PEDERSON, A., BABIGAN, H., IZZO, L., & TROST, M. (1973). Long term followup of early detected vulnerable children. *Journal of Consulting and Clinical Psychology, 41,* 438-446.

DWIGGINS, D. (1981). *An investigation of differences in teacher standards and expectations that teachers hold for handicapped versus nonhandicapped students.* Unpublished doctoral dissertation, University of Oregon, Eugene, Oregon.

FREDERICKS, H. D. B., BALDWIN, V., GROVE, D., MOORE, W., RIGGS, C., & LYONS, B. (1978). Integrating the moderately and severely handicapped preschool child into a normal day care setting. In M. Guralnick (Ed.), *Early intervention and the integration of handicapped and nonhandicapped children.* Baltimore: University Park Press.

GOTTLIEB, J. (1978). Observing social adaptation in schools. In G. Sackett (Ed.), *Observing behavior (Vol. I): Theory and applications in mental retardation.* Baltimore: University Park Press.

GOTTLIEB, J. (1979). Placement in the least restrictive environment. In *LRE: Developing criteria for the evaluation of the least restrictive environment provision.* Philadelphia: Research for Better Schools.

GOTTLIEB, J., & BUDOFF, M. (1973). Social acceptability of retarded children in nongraded schools differing in architecture. *American Journal of Mental Deficiency, 78,* 15-19.

GOTTMAN, J. (1977). Toward a definition of social isolation in children. *Child Development, 48,* 513-517.

GOTTMAN, J., GONSO, J., & RASMUSSEN, B. (1975). Social interaction, social competence, and friendship in children. *Child Development, 46,* 709-718.

GOTTMAN, J., GONSO, J., & SCHULER, P. (1976). Teaching social skills to isolated children.

Child Development, 4, 179-197.

GREENWOOD, C. R., HOPS, H., & WALKER, H. M. (1977). The durability of student behavior change. *Behavior Therapy, 8,* 631-638.

GREENWOOD, C. R., TODD, N. M., HOPS, H., & WALKER, H. M. (1982). Behavior change targets in the assessment and treatment of socially withdrawn preschool children. *Behavioral Assessment, 4,* 237-297.

GREENWOOD, C. R., WALKER, H. M., TODD, N. M., & HOPS, H. (1979). *SAMPLE: Social Assessment Manual for Preschool LEvel.* Center at Oregon for Research in the Behavioral Education of the Handicapped (CORBEH), University of Oregon, Eugene, Oregon.

GREENWOOD, C. R., WALKER, H. M., TODD, N. M., & HOPS, H. (1981). Normative and descriptive analysis of preschool free play social interaction rates. *Journal of Pediatric Psychology, 6,* 343-367.

GRESHAM, F. (1981). Social skills training with handicapped children: A review. *Review of Educational Research, 51*(1), 139-176.

GRESHAM, F. (1982). Misguided mainstreaming: The case for social skills training with handicapped children. *Exceptional Children, 48,* 422-433.

GRONLUND, N. E., & ANDERSON, L. (1957). Personality characteristics of socially accepted, socially neglected, and socially rejected junior high pupils. *Educational Administration and Supervision, 43,* 329-338.

GURALNICK, M. (1978). Integrated preschools as educational and therapeutic environments. In M. Guralnick (Ed.), *Early intervention and the integration of handicapped and nonhandicapped children.* Baltimore: University Park Press.

GURALNICK, M. (1981). Programmatic factors affecting child-child social interactions in mainstreamed preschool program. *Exceptional Education Quarterly, 1,* 71-91.

HARTUP, W. (1979). Peer relations and the growth of social competence. In M. W. Kent & J. E. Rolf (Eds.), *Primary prevention of psychopathology (Vol. 3): Social competence in children.* Hanover, NH: University Press of New England.

HERSH, R., & WALKER, H. M. (1983). Great expectations: Making schools effective for all children. *Policy Studies Review, 2,* 147-188.

HOGE, R. D., & LUCE, S. (1979). Predicting academic achievement from classroom behavior. *Review of Educational Research, 49,* 479-496.

HOPS, H. (in press). Social skills training for socially withdrawn/isolated children. In P. Karoly & J. Steffen (Eds.), *Enhancing children's competencies.* Lexington, MA: Lexington Books.

HOPS, H., & FINCH, M. (1981, May). *A skill deficit view of social competence in preschoolers.* Paper presented at the meeting of the Association for Behavior Analysis, Milwaukee.

HOPS, H., WALKER, H. M., & GREENWOOD, C. R. (1979). PEERS. A program for remediating social withdrawal in school: Behavioral systems for the developmentally disabled. In L. A. Hamerlynck (Ed.), *Behavioral systems for the developmentally disabled: School and family environments.* New York: Brunner/Mazel.

IANO, R. P., AYERS, D., HELLER, H. B., McGETTIGAN, J. F., & WALKER, V. S. (1974). Sociometric status of retarded children in an integrative program. *Exceptional Children, 40,* 267-271.

KAZDIN, A. (1977). Assessing the clinical or applied importance of behavior change through social validation. *Behavior Modification, 4,* 427-452.

KEOGH, B., & LEVITT, M. (1976). Special education in the mainstream: A confrontation of limitations. *Focus on Exceptional Children, 8,* 1-10.

KORNBLAU, B., & KEOGH, B. (1980). Teachers' perceptions and educational decisions. *Journal of Teaching and Learning, 1,* 87-101.

LADD, C. W. (1981). Social skills and peer acceptance: Effects of a social learning method for training social skills. *Child Development, 52,* 171-178.

LaGRECA, A., & SANTOGROSSI, D. (1980). Social skills training with elementary school students: A behavioral group approach. *Journal of Consulting and Clinical Psychology, 48,* 220-227.

LARRIVEE, B., & COOK, L. (1979). Mainstreaming: A study of the variables affecting teacher attitude. *Journal of Special Education, 13,* 315-324.

LOWENBRAUN, S., & AFFLECK, J. O. (1979). Least restrictive environment. In *LRE: Developing criteria for the evaluation of the least restrictive environment provision.* Philadelphia: Research for Better Schools.

LYNN, L. E., Jr. (1981). The emerging system for educating handicapped children. *Policy Studies Review, 2,* 21-58.

MacMILLAN, D. L., & MORRISON, G. M. (1980). Correlates of social status among mildly handicapped learners in self-contained special classes. *Journal of Educational Psychology, 72,* 437-444.

McCONNELL, S. (1982, May). *Experimental validation of the ACCEPTS social skills curriculum.* Paper presented at the meeting of the Association for Behavior Analysis, Milwaukee.

O'CONNOR, R.D. (1969). Modification of social withdrawal through symbolic modeling. *Journal of Applied Behavior Analysis, 2,* 15-22.

ODEN, S., & ASHER, S. (1977). Coaching children in social skills for friendship making. *Child Development, 48,* 495-506.

O'LEARY, S. G., & O'LEARY, K. D. (1976). Behavior modification in the school. In H. Leitenberg (Ed.), *Handbook of behavior modification.* Englewood Cliffs, NJ: Prentice-Hall.

PECK, C. A., COOKE, T. P., & APOLLONI, T. (1981). Utilization of peer imitation in therapeutic and instructional contexts. In P. S. Strain (Ed.), *The utilization of classroom peers as behavior change agents.* New York: Plenum.

ROBINS, L. (1966). *Deviant children grown up.* Baltimore: William & Wilkins.

ROFF, M. (1961). Childhood social interactions and young adult bad conduct. *Journal of Abnormal Social Psychology, 63,* 333-337.

ROFF, M., SELLS, B., & GOLDEN, M. (1972). *Social adjustment and personality development in children.* Minneapolis: University of Minnesota Press.

ROGERS-WARREN, A., & WARREN, S. (1977). *Ecological perspectives in behavior analysis.* Baltimore: University Park Press.

VAN LIESHOUT, C. F. M. (1973, August). *The assessment of stability and change in peer interaction of normal hearing and deaf preschool children.* Paper presented at the meeting of the International Society for the Study of Behavioral Development, Ann Arbor, Michigan.

WALKER, H. M. (1984). The SBS program (Social Behavior Survival): A systematic approach to the integration of handicapped children into less restrictive settings. *Education and Treatment of Children, 6*(4), 421.

WALKER, H. M., & HOPS, H. (1976). Use of normative peer data as a standard for evaluating classroom treatment effects. *Journal of Applied Behavior Analysis, 9,* 159-168.

WALKER, H. M., McCONNELL, S., HOLMES, D., TODIS, B., WALKER, J., & GOLDEN, N. (1983). *The Walker social skills curriculum: The ACCEPTS program.* Austin: PRO-ED.

WALKER, H. M., McCONNELL, S., WALKER, J., CLARKE, J., TODIS, B., COHEN, G., & RANKIN, R. (1983). Initial analysis of the ACCEPTS curriculum: Efficacy of instructional and behavior management procedures for improving the social competence of handicapped children. *Analysis and Intervention in Developmental Disabilities, 3,* 105-127.

WALKER, H. M., & RANKIN, R. (1983). Assessing the behavioral expectations and demands of less restrictive settings: Instruments, ecological assessment procedures, and outcomes. In R. Martin (Ed.), *Social Psychology Review, 12,* 274-284.

ZAX, M., COWEN, E., RAPPAPORT, J., BEACH, D., & LAIRD, J. (1968). Followup study of children identified early as emotionally disturbed. *Journal of Consulting Psychology, 32,* 369-373.

8

Childhood Autism: Developmental Considerations and Behavioral Interventions by Professionals, Families, and Peers

WILLIAM R. JENSON and K. RICHARD YOUNG

Autism has had a varied and controversial history. As early as 1799, there were reports of children who were wild and raised by animals. Victor, the Wild Boy of Aveyron (Itard, 1962), who was found wandering the woods, was most likely an autistic boy. It was assumed at the time that Victor had been raised by wolves, but it is most likely he was abandoned or lost by parents who could not cope with the strange rocking behavior, lack of language, poor attention, and inappropriate social behaviors that he exhibited. It was not until 144 years later that Dr. Leo Kanner (1943) recognized autism as a distinctive psychiatric condition. In the 11 autistic children that Kanner studied, he identified the following characteristics: failure to develop socially, disrupted language, an intense need to maintain the environment with no changes (sameness), self-stimulatory behavior such as hand flapping or twirling, and a fascination or fear of mechanical objects. Kanner mistakenly believed that autistic children had normal intelligence and it was their failure to relate socially that precluded normal development and social interaction.

Perhaps the most controversial aspect in the history of autism is the speculation that the cause of social withdrawal and other autistic characteristics is cold, rejecting, overintellectual parents, particularly mothers (King, 1975; Reiser & Brown, 1964). The term "schizophrenogenic mother" was coined to describe a perfectionist, cold, and rejecting mother who caused autism. Few professionals now believe that parents cause autism. Excellent scientific evidence indicates a genetic (Folstein & Rutter, 1978) or viral (Chess, 1977) etiology.

During the past 40 years, scientific research has made major advances in the treatment and study of autistic children. In the 1970s alone there were over 1,100 publications on autism—a threefold increase from the previous decade (DeMyer, Hingtgen, & Jackson, 1981). Autism was previously considered to be a psychotic condition, where a child developed normally and then withdrew into a psychotic state; but today it is defined as a developmental disability in which the child has never developed appropriate social, language, and adaptive skills. A great deal is now known about autistic persons' development from childhood through their adult life. Most importantly, an enormous research effort devoted to the treatment of autistic persons is reducing the rate of institutionalization. The focus of this chapter is the description and developmental characteristics of autistic persons and the treatment procedures that have been experimentally validated. Emphasis is placed on the behavior therapy approach to treatment, particularly the use of standardized core management programs that utilize professional staff, volunteers, families, and peers in the treatment process.

IDENTIFICATION AND CLASSIFICATION OF AUTISM

The field of autism has lacked professional agreement on a definition and appropriate identification procedures. However, in the past five years definitions of infantile autism have become more standardized (Rutter, 1978a; Schopler, 1978). The American Psychiatric Association has included autism in the Diagnostic and Statistical Manual of Mental Disorders for the first time (American Psychiatric Association, 1980). The DSM-III diagnostic criteria for autism include:

1) Onset before 30 months;

2) Pervasive lack of responsiveness to other people (autism);
3) Gross deficits in language development;
4) If speech is present, peculiar speech patterns such as immediate and delayed echolalia, metaphorical language, pronominal reversal;
5) Bizarre responses to various aspects of the environment; e.g., resistance to change, peculiar interest or attachments to animate or inanimate objects;
6) Absence of delusions, hallucinations, loosening of associations, and incoherence as in schizophrenia. (pp. 89-90)

The DSM-III definition of autism emphasizes an early onset of the condition and disturbed social interactions. Similarly, the National Society for Autistic Children and Adults (NSAC, 1978) defines autism as an early onset condition and emphasizes delayed development in three major areas: motor, social-adaptive, and cognitive functioning. NSAC lists several problem areas including 1) irregular responses to sensory stimuli, 2) communication difficulties (speech, language-cognition, and nonverbal communication), and 3) inability to relate appropriately to people, events, and objects. Characteristics such as self-stimulation or self-injury, inappropriate giggling and laughter, lack of an appreciation of real danger, and mental retardation are also commonly associated with autism. The NSAC definition points out that a majority of autistic children (60–70%) are also mentally retarded.

Although the DSM-III and NSAC definitions of autism have improved the agreement among professionals, the definition is still broad and often difficult to apply in specific cases. This is especially true since there is a distinct overlap between autism and other conditions such as mental retardation or hyperactivity and symptoms are often not particularly clear. In such cases, an objective behavior checklist is helpful in identifying behavioral symptoms. A number of autism behavior checklists are available. In the past, one of the most commonly used instruments has been the Rimland E-2 checklist. This checklist, however, has been criticized for questionable reliability, its limited ability to differentiate between autism and mental retardation, and questionable criterion validity (DeMyer et al., 1981). Two other common rating instruments include the Behavior Rating Instrument for Autistic and Atypical Children (BRIAAC) developed by Cohen, Caparulo, Gold, Waldo, Shaywitz, Ruttenberg, and Rimland (1978), and the Childhood Autism Rating Scale (CARS) developed by Schopler, Reichler, DeVillis, and Daly (1980). One of the most promising autism checklists is the Autism Behavior Checklist (ABC) (Krug, Arick, &

Almond, 1979). This checklist has excellent reliability and criterion validity. The ABC checklist identified in its standardization group 90% of the children who had an independent diagnosis of autism.

Standardized behavior checklists for autistic children are an improvement over a clinician's judgment based on broad guidelines such as the DSM-III or NSAC definitions of autism. However, even specific behavior checklists do not cover all of the points of comparison needed for assessing and classifying autistic children. The Autism Decision Matrix (Jenson & Reavis, 1982) was designed to incorporate information from autism behavior checklists, recognized classification descriptions (DSM-III), and previous research findings to reach a diagnostic decision for individual cases (see Figure 1). Existing checklists, such as the Autism Behavior Checklist or the E-2, are utilized and, if possible, completed by both a parent and a teacher. The cutoff scores from the checklists are then listed in three columns: A—indicating the child is on or above the cutoff score, B—indicating questionable diagnosis, or C—indicating the child is well below the cutoff score. The matrix manual guides a clinician or teacher through a series of steps that examine the following factors: social relatedness, language variables, self-stimulation and self-injury variables, the need for sameness, age of onset, intelligence, and autism as differentiated from childhood schizophrenia. The factors in each step of the comparison were selected from and substantiated by research. They are written in simple terms so that a professional who is not familiar with the area of autism can easily make the comparisons. The Autism Decision Matrix shows promise as an instrument that can facilitate the diagnosis of autism. However, more research is needed regarding reliability and validity characteristics.

DEVELOPMENTAL AND BEHAVIORAL CHARACTERISTICS OF AUTISM

Not all autistic children exhibit all of the symptoms discussed or all of those included in the classification systems. The behavioral symptoms occur on a continuum, both in terms of the number of characteristics a child may demonstrate and the severity of the problems. Not only do the presence and severity of symptoms differ from child to child, but they also may change as the child grows and develops.

	A	B	C

Step #1
  Parent's Checklist
  Teacher's Checklist			

Step #2 Social Relatedness			
Step #3 Language			
Step #4 Self-stimulation or Injury			
Step #5 Sameness			
Step #6 Age of Onset			
Step #7 Intelligence			
Step #8 Autism vs. Schizophrenia			
SUM			
Other Considerations: 1. No fear of danger			
2. Aggression, temper tantrum, noncompliance			
3. Adaptive behavior training needed			

FIGURE 1. Autism Decision Matrix (Jenson & Reavis, 1982)

Social Development

   Possibly one of the most difficult behaviors to define and assess is
"social relatedness." The inability to relate socially to other human
beings frequently becomes the primary diagnostic consideration in determining if a child is "truly" autistic. However, a concise definition
of "social relatedness" is lacking, and the research that has been done
on social relatedness is not as objective as other research in the field
of autism. Some of the behaviors that have been described as part of
social relatedness include: gaze aversion, inappropriate laughter, social
avoidance, poor modeling skills, social aloofness, passive interaction,
and poor play skills. None of these behaviors alone necessarily indicates poor social relatedness, but some combination of such variables
can lead to total social isolation. Other factors such as language skills
(Wing & Gould, 1979), intelligence, and perceptual discrimination
skills (Schreibman & Lovaas, 1973) may also affect the autistic child's
social abilities.
   Some of the research that has been conducted on social relatedness
has investigated eye contact and gaze aversion. Hutt and Ounsted
(1970) found that autistic children were less likely than normal children to draw pictures of faces that included eyes. When autistic children are picked up by adults, they typically turn away and avoid eye
contact. Gaze aversion and poor eye contact, however, can be effectively
changed through behavioral intervention procedures, such as shaping
with use of edible reinforcers and overcorrection procedures (Foxx,
1977). Research has demonstrated that autistic children have a lower
avoidance threshold regarding the approach of other people than do
normal children (Richer, 1978). In particular, autistic children are
more likely to avoid people who stare, smile, or attempt to establish
eye contact when approaching (Richer, 1978; Richer & Richards, 1975).
Social avoidance can also be reduced through behavioral interventions
(Lovaas, Schaeffer, & Simmons, 1965; Romanczyk, Diamant, Goren,
Trunell, & Harris, 1975) and the use of peers as models (Ragland, Kerr,
& Strain, 1978; Stainback & Stainback, 1982; Strain, Kerr, & Ragland,
1979).
   Although general improvement with autistic children can be made
in the areas of eye contact and social interactions, research has shown
that generalization and maintenance of these behaviors is difficult to
obtain and requires special programming (Ragland et al., 1978; Strain
et al., 1979). To date, the social problems exhibited by autistic individuals can only be managed and improved; they cannot be entirely

eliminated, and appear to be part of an autistic person's development from childhood through adult life. Social relationships such as marriage or having children are extremely rare in autistic adults.

The developmental basis for the lack of social responsiveness in autistic children is not clearly understood, but it seems that the problem is a failure to develop normal social abilities, rather than a loss of previously learned skills. Some researchers have observed a phenomenon they have labeled the "autistic circle" (Manzano & Pralong, 1982) which is, in effect, a precisely defined area around an autistic child in which he or she will approach and pay attention to objects. However, if an object is placed outside of the circle, the child will not show interest in it. This autistic circle of interest may have a critical effect on the child's development. For example, if during the period of initial social development an autistic child will not respond to people because they are outside his or her circle, then valuable opportunities to develop social relatedness are lost. Data on the autistic circle of interest are extremely limited and more research is needed. The phenomenon may be related to what has been called a critical developmental period.

Hayden and McGinness (1977) have suggested that there are critical periods for the development of certain skills, and a failure to capitalize on those periods may result in serious developmental deficiencies. Research with animals has shown critical periods for social development (Harlow & Harlow, 1971). The research demonstrated that social deprivation at a young age profoundly affects the later development of social skills. Although it is basically speculation at this point, autistic children may also fail to develop socially during a critical period. The consequence is a lack of social abilities, which leads to social avoidance, which in turn may partially deprive them of the social stimulation needed to develop appropriate socialization skills. More research is needed in this area, particularly research that focuses on periods critical to social development.

Language Development

Language disturbances are common in a large majority of autistic children. Many autistic children are totally mute, in that they use no verbal forms of communication. Other autistic children may demonstrate echolalia, pronoun reversals (e.g., you for I), difficulty in discrimination of polar language concepts (such as yes and no), and a profound difficulty in understanding language. The development of language in autistic children is delayed and markedly deviant once it appears (Rutter, 1978b). Prelanguage skills that are evident in normal children are absent in autistic children. For example, many autistic children do not babble as normal children do prior to learning more advanced language skills (Bartak, Rutter, & Cox, 1975). The imitation of gestures and verbal stimuli is another critical prerequisite to language that is absent from the autistic child's behavioral repertoire.

Perhaps the autistic child's greatest language difficulty is the lack of comprehension. Language is an abstract symbol system that permits the communication of messages (Paluszny, 1979), and autistic children have difficulty in dealing with abstract concepts. During the first year of life normal children learn to understand a great deal and even though they speak few, if any, words, they learn to communicate with gestures. Autistic children fail to develop this understanding and ability to communicate. They often completely lack communication skills and have very poor receptive language. Abstract terms and phrases are very difficult for autistic children, in that they are likely to interpret word meanings literally or concretely rather than abstractly (Rutter, 1974). This lack of language comprehension may also produce other types of language problems, such as echolalia, which further disrupts the language development.

The delay in normal language development, and its abnormal characteristics once it appears, is not likely a function of hearing deficits or motivational problems (Rutter, 1974). Rather, the language problems appear to be a result of cognitive deficits and perceptual problems. Long-term follow-up studies have shown that the more severely intellectually affected autistic children were, the more likely they were to develop speech and language problems (Rutter, Greenfield, & Lockyer, 1967). Autistic children respond poorly on the performance subtests of the Wechsler Intelligence Test for Children that have high verbal loadings, even when these subtests do not require the use of speech (Rutter, 1978b). Perceptual difficulties (e.g., stimulus overselectivity) are also related to poor language acquisition in autistic children, who commonly have more difficulty in processing auditory information than visual information. Combined sign language and verbal language presentations (total communication) have been successful in increasing verbal language in some autistic children (Carr, 1979). Sign language has been used as a visual cue in teaching autistic children difficult verbal language discriminations, such as "Yes" and "No" discriminations (Walker, Hinerman, Jenson, & Petersen, 1981) and verbally discriminating between different colors (Van Wagenen, Jenson, Worsham, & Petersen, 1983).

Most autistic children have severe comprehension and expressive language difficulties throughout their lives. About half of autistic adults do not have useful speech which greatly impacts on their social adjustment. Rutter (1978b) has noted that even the autistic children who developed near-normal levels of language competence still had speech and language abnormalities as adults. Common problems included perseverative or obsessive question asking, speech that was monotonous and lacking in inflection, and difficulties with language abstractions.

Intellectual Functioning

Intellectual deficits are part of the autism syndrome with particular difficulties occurring in skills that require verbal abilities. Rutter (1970) estimates that two-thirds to three-fourths of all autistic persons will suffer from mental retardation throughout their lives. DeMyer, Barton, Alpern, Kimberlin, Allen, Yang, and Steele (1974) found that 74% of the autistic children they tested had IQ scores below 52 and only 2.6% had scores above 85. Most of these children scored higher on the "performance" subtests than on the "verbal" subtests of intelligence tests. As mentioned earlier, some autistic children appear to have normal or superior abilities in some intellectual areas such as mathematical skills, musical abilities, calculation of calendar dates, or artistic abilities. These splinter skills are generally accompanied by retardation of other skills (Creak, 1961) and they do not significantly influence the child's overall IQ scores (DeMyer et al., 1981). Only about 10% of autistic children (Rimland, 1978) show these splinter skills, but they present a problem because they often lead to an overestimation of an autistic child's intellectual ability.

The intellectual retardation of autistic children appears to be very stable over time, and does not change even with improvements in other areas. Lockyer and Rutter (1969) reported that the IQ scores of autistic persons did not change significantly over a 10-year period even when there were improvements in social relationships with other people.

Stimulus Overselectivity

Difficulties with visual and verbal discriminations are profound handicaps that an autistic child faces in learning to adjust to a normal environment. These discrimination difficulties are frequently related to a phenomenon labeled *stimulus overselectivity* (Lovaas, Schreibman,

Koegel, & Rehm, 1971). Essentially, stimulus overselectivity is a perceptual disability in which a child responds "only to part of a relevant cue, or even to a minor, often irrelevant feature of the environment, without learning about other portions of the environment" (Lovaas, Koegel, & Schreibman, 1979). For example, an autistic child may learn to discriminate male and female dolls only by looking at the differences in their shoes and when the shoes are changed the discrimination breaks down (Schreibman & Lovaas, 1973). Normal children, in learning a sex discrimination between dolls, used a number of cues to form the discrimination, particularly the features of the doll's head. Autistic children used irrelevant cues, such as the shoes, and consistently avoided using the doll's head to form their discrimination.

Stimulus overselectivity can affect social interactions, language development, the use of imitation skills, and generalization of newly learned skills to nontraining conditions. Overselectivity has been exhibited by a large number of autistic children (Lovaas et al., 1979) and other children as well, including mentally retarded children (Lovaas et al., 1971), learning disabled children (Bailey, 1981), and normal children (Schover & Newsom, 1976) and has a severe and debilitating effect on the learning of the child. Overselectivity occurs between different types of stimulus modalities, such as auditory and visual stimuli; i.e., a child prefers one modality to the exclusion of the other. It also occurs within a modality: A child prefers one stimulus dimension over another, such as loud sounds over soft sounds. Overselectivity is related to IQ level, with the most severe forms of overselectivity exhibited by autistic children with the greatest degree of mental retardation (Wilhelm & Lovaas, 1976). From a developmental perspective, overselectivity is related to the chronological age of the child. Younger autistic children are more likely to show overselectivity than older autistic children (Schover & Newsom, 1976). It is interesting to note that some normal children also appear to go through an overselectivity stage, but the normal children who show visual overselectivity appear to be far ahead of their autistic counterparts in emotional, social, linguistic, and intellectual abilities (Schover & Newsom, 1976). Normal children move out of the overselectivity stage, while autistic children continue to be handicapped by it. Similarly, overselectivity may also be responsible for the "need for sameness" characteristic that is found in so many autistic children. Autistic children may memorize or use irrelevant cues in their environments to adjust and function. When minor changes are made in furniture arrangements, time schedules, or ritualistic procedures, the autistic child may lose these cues or points of reference and react by throwing tantrums.

Self-stimulation and Self-injury

Self-stimulation is commonly exhibited by autistic children in such forms as rocking, gazing at objects and lights, rhythmic manipulation of objects, and/or hand flapping. It is common for nonhandicapped persons, both children and adults, to occasionally engage in some form of self-stimulation; e.g., foot wiggling, hair stroking, nail biting. The basic difference is that autistic children exhibit high rates of self-stimulation and usually in much more exaggerated forms. Self-stimulation serves no apparent purpose other than sensory input, but the effects can be deleterious to autistic children because this activity totally absorbs the child's attention. Research has shown that self-stimulation in autistic children interferes with gaining the child's attention and, therefore, learning new responses (Koegel & Covert, 1972). It also interferes with observational learning (Varni, Lovaas, Koegel, & Everett, 1979) and appropriate play (Koegel, Firestone, Kramme, & Dunlap, 1974). Self-stimulation is partially a function of the child's level of intelligence and of the amount and quality of stimulation in the child's environment. Frankel, Freeman, Ritvo, and Pardo (1978) found that autistic children with higher IQ scores had lower rates of self-stimulation in complex and stimulating environments and higher rates of self-stimulation in low-stimulation environments. The effects were the opposite for autistic children with low IQs. The reinforcing qualities of self-stimulation may be tied to the sensory feedback provided by the self-stimulation behavior. For example, Devany and Rincover (1982) demonstrated that by removing sensory feedback (sensory extinction), self-stimulatory behaviors such as finger flapping, object twirling, and light switching could be reduced.

Self-injury is similar to self-stimulation except that it does not occur in as many autistic persons. Researchers estimate that from five (Frankel & Simmons, 1976) to 10% (Schroeder, Schroeder, Smith, & Dalldorf, 1978) of the autistic population engage in self-injurious behavior. Common forms of self-injurious behavior include head banging, eye gouging, face hitting, biting, and mouthing. Like self-stimulation, self-injury is related to the intellectual level of the autistic child and to the sensory feedback characteristics (Rincover, 1981) associated with the behavior. Autistic children with lower IQs are more likely to engage in self-injurious behavior than children with near normal IQs (Bartak & Rutter, 1976). Self-injurious behavior may be reinforced by helping the autistic child escape or avoid tasks and/or requests from adults (Carr, 1977; Carr, Newsom, & Binkoff, 1976). In fact, restraints that are used to prevent self-injury have been observed to develop reinforcing characteristics because they restrict the person from having to comply with a number of demands made by the environment. Researchers have used access to restraints as a reinforcer for not engaging in self-injurious behavior while the patient is out of restraints (Favell, McGimsey, & Jones, 1978).

Self-stimulation and self-injury have been shown to be related to the age and the development of the child. Wolff (1967) speculated that self-stimulation is a valuable part of a child's motor development. According to Wolff, normal children pass through this stage of development. He hypothesizes that due to neurological deficits, retarded and psychotic children often do not pass through this stage. Carr (1982) has pointed out that a number of normal children (nine to 17%) engage in self-injurious behavior at very young ages (nine to 32 months of age), especially head banging. Schroeder et al. (1978) found that younger patients had higher frequencies of self-injurious behavior, particularly if they had deficits in intellectual functioning, vision, or language disorders.

LONG-TERM DEVELOPMENT AND PROGNOSIS

Autism is a life-long condition with a very consistent and stable course. Unlike other psychotic conditions, which may vacillate from greatly improved states to severely affected states, autism is stable from childhood through adult life, even though individuals make limited improvements through therapeutic intervention. Longitudinal studies done in the 1950s through the 1970s reported that five to 17% of autistic children had good outcomes, while 60 to 70% generally had poor outcomes (Lotter, 1978; DeMyer, Barton, DeMyer, Norton, Allen, & Steele, 1973). In 1971, Kanner stated that approximately half of all autistic children were institutionalized, and once institutionalized very few were released.

Two powerful predictive variables for long-term prognosis for autistic children are intelligence and language. For example, an IQ score below 50 indicates poor prognosis regardless of other variables. If the child's

IQ score is near normal and there is only a mild language disorder, then the prognosis is good (Rutter, 1974). Although both language and IQ scores are useful indicators in predicting an autistic child's adjustment, they are still only gross indicators. Other variables that are important include early intervention and the inclusion of parents as part of the treatment team. Lovaas, Koegel, Simmons, and Long (1973) have shown that a parent's willingness to be trained and to use strong consequences for their child's behavior are very important variables in determining whether the child will be institutionalized or function in a community/home setting.

One of the most impressive demonstrations of early interventions involved parents as part of the treatment process. The Division for the Treatment and Education of Autistic and Related Communication Handicapped Children (TEACCH) of the University of North Carolina has operated a statewide treatment and education program for autistic persons since 1972, and has reduced institutionalization to only 8% of the autistic population. These results underscore the need for early intervention and the training of parents and families.

BEHAVIORAL INTERVENTIONS WITH AUTISTIC CHILDREN

The remainder of this chapter will review behavioral intervention strategies that have been proven effective in the treatment of autistic children. Particular attention will be given to parent and peer interventions and programs developed by the authors. Behavior therapy conducted in one-to-one teaching situations has been responsible for much of the success achieved in the treatment of autistic children. This approach has been used to teach generalized imitation (Lovaas, Freitas, Nelson, & Whalen, 1967), functional speech (Lovaas, 1977), conversational speech (Lovaas, 1966), appropriate play skills (Koegel et al., 1974), reading (Hewitt, 1964), self-help skills (Marshall, 1966), and to eliminate inappropriate behaviors (Koegel & Covert, 1972). Although autistic children are not completely cured by these treatments, significant advances have been made in teaching autistic children new skills and in managing inappropriate behaviors (Lovaas & Bucher, 1974; Koegel, Rincover, & Egel, 1982). In spite of the success of these treatments, there are major disadvantages in the use of one-to-one interventions; i.e., difficulties in generalizing treatment gains and the cost and time involved in providing treatment. Consistently staffing

many different individual behavior therapy programs can be a night-
mare for a teacher or clinician who is responsible for a number of
autistic children.

The use of discrete trials is a standard approach to the treatment of
autistic persons and has been the basis of most behavioral interventions (Donnellan, Gossage, LaVigna, Schuler, & Traphagen, 1977;
Koegel, Schreibman, Britten, Burke, & O'Neill, 1982). Essentially, a
discrete trial consists of 1) a clear beginning (signaled by a discriminative stimulus) and ending of a trial, 2) a behaviorally defined standard (observable and measurable) to judge a behavior, 3) a consequence
for the behavior, and 4) an intertrial interval of very short duration
(three to five seconds) in which no teaching occurs and data are recorded. A series of prompts can be used with discrete trials to initially
shape a behavior, although these prompts are generally faded out.

At the Children's Behavior Therapy Unit (CBTU), in Salt Lake City,
Utah, we use the discrete trial format in our "core management" programs (Jenson & CBTU Staff, 1980). The programs are used with *all*
autistic children at the school to shape 1) attending (Get Ready Program), 2) following directions from adults, 3) visual tracking (an advanced attending program), 4) motor and verbal imitation, and 5) other
basic instructional programs. Each child goes through the core management programs at their own speed depending on their abilities and
intelligence. Since data are recorded during each intertrial interval,
the child's success can be calculated each day and modifications can
be made if necessary. Each core management program follows a task
analysis format, sequencing steps from the very simple to more complex. Each program acts as a criterion-referenced test in that a child
must be at least 80% correct across 40 trials before being allowed to
advance to the next step in the program.

The child is reinforced after each correct trial with an edible or
preferred reinforcer which is paired with a social reinforcer (e.g., a hug
or tickle from the therapist). The concept behind pairing social interaction with an edible reinforcer is to build the social interaction as a
conditioned reinforcer and break down the "social nonrelatedness" of
the autistic child. Later in the program, social reinforcement replaces
the edible or other artificial reinforcers. If a child responds incorrectly,
the therapist looks away for five seconds (an extinction procedure). If
the child misbehaves, a mild "stand-up, sit-down" form of contingent
exercise or overcorrection is used to decrease the inappropriate behavior. After each 30-minute session, the therapists and settings are

changed. This reduces dependency on one adult or setting and the child's insistence on "sameness." All instructions are given using total communication (signs and verbal words). All the core management programs are designed to develop instructional control and increase the child's ability to be taught in a more cost-effective group format.

The "Get Ready Attending Program" is the first core management program taught. This program teaches the autistic child to sit in a chair and attend to a therapist without self-stimulating or being noncompliant. In a discrete trial format, the child is taught to sit in a chair, with his feet on the floor, hands in his lap, and to make eye contact. A prompt-fading sequence is used in which the therapist first holds the child's feet (full physical prompt), then fades the prompt after a number of successful trials to touching the child's feet (partial physical prompt), then to pointing to the child's feet (partial prompt), and then finally to having the child's feet on the floor with the verbal prompt, "Get Ready." After the "feet on floor" response is taught, the therapist concentrates on "hands in the lap" and later eye contact using the same shaping sequence. The discriminative stimuli are used to signal correct responding, establish instructional control over the child's behavior, and can be used as a tool in other treatment programs. For example, giving the instruction "Get Ready" may be used to stop tantrums in nontraining settings or to gain the child's attention when working on other more complex tasks. Similarly, the "Following Directions Program" teaches an autistic child to respond to common adult requests. This simplifies administering the "stand-up/sit-down" overcorrection procedure because the child follows verbal instructions. All core management programs including the "Following Directions Program" utilize the same basic prompting and fading sequence as the "Get Ready Attending Program."

All of the core management programs are designed to give maximum instructional control to the therapist and/or parent. Since each program is written in a step-by-step sequence, they are easily used in clinics, classrooms, and as a base for training parents, siblings, or peers. The standardized nature of the programs allows autistic children to be treated in a systematic fashion by different therapists, as well as students and volunteers. All core management programs selectively reinforce attending, compliance and language skills, which are incompatible with self-stimulation or self-injury. Each program is criterion-referenced so that no child is held back, but advances at his or her own speed. The programs are simple enough that a seven-year-old peer can run any core management program successfully. This simplicity adds greatly in the generalized use of the programs by parents, siblings, and normal peers in various classroom and community settings.

PARENT TRAINING

As mentioned above, behavior modification programs with autistic children have resulted in positive treatment gains. These programs typically involve one-to-one teaching situations and require large expenditures of time and effort (Koegel et al., 1982). If one-to-one instruction is provided by professional therapists it is also very costly. The costs are further compounded by the failure of autistic children to generalize skills taught from one-to-one instruction by the therapist to other settings and persons, and the failure of skill maintenance over time. Egel (1982) has pointed out that the lack of generalization and maintenance places severe limitations on autistic children as they encounter many different persons, settings, and stimuli.

As a solution to both of these problems (substantial time and effort in training autistic children and the frequent failure of the results of training to maintain and generalize), there is an increasing trend by researchers and service providers to involve parents in the treatment process (Freeman & Ritvo, 1976; Koegel, Glahn, & Nieminen, 1978; Lovaas et al., 1973; Nordquist & Wahler, 1973; Schopler & Reichler, 1971). Lovaas et al. (1973) compared autistic children who had been treated in a clinic without parental involvement to autistic children whose parents were trained to conduct therapy. They found that parent training and involvement resulted in more durable treatment gains. They further suggested that parental involvement aids generalization to nontraining conditions.

Koegel et al. (1978) trained parents to use a discrete trial format to instruct their autistic children. Parents were taught by modeling, videotapes, and practice to present discriminative stimuli and to use prompts, shaping, and consequences. The results demonstrated that parents could reliably use the procedures to improve the behavior of autistic children after training but not before.

Koegel et al. (1982) summarized the results of a series of comprehensive parent training studies. They concluded that parent training produced better initial improvement and more durable treatment effects than clinic groups and was superior to clinic treatment because the treatment was presented in many different settings. Psychological and marital adjustment measures did not reveal any problems for parents involved in the treatment program.

The results of the research and training efforts clearly indicate that parents can be trained as competent therapists for autistic children and that their involvement in the treatment process may be critical to initial and long-term behavioral improvements. A note of caution is warranted by the suggestion of Nordquist and Wahler (1973) that parents must "comprehend the extent of their commitment, many months of continuous treatment may be required to obtain treatment results" (p. 86). Lovaas et al. (1973) stated that not all parents may be equally successful as therapists. They pointed out that parents must be willing to use strong consequences, treat the child as if he or she can succeed, and commit a major part of their lives to the autistic child. However, parents can play a critical role in the treatment of their autistic children, without necessarily creating adverse effects on the family or marital relationships (Koegel et al., 1982).

PEER INVOLVEMENT

Peers are another excellent resource for use in treatment programs with autistic children. Peers have been successfully utilized in a variety of programs with severely handicapped persons. Gladstone and Sherman (1975) taught nonhandicapped high school students to correctly use verbal instructions, physical prompts, reinforcement, and ignoring in teaching institutionalized profoundly retarded children (ages six to 14) to follow simple directions. Peer tutors have been used to teach mentally retarded students object recognition, shape discrimination, taking off clothes, rolling a ball, and climbing stairs (Fenrick & McDonnell, 1980), vocal imitation (Raver et al., 1978), free play behavior (Peck et al., 1978), playground skills (Donder & Nietupski, 1981), and leisure time skills (Hill & Wehman, 1980).

Peer tutors have also been used with autistic children. Ragland et al. (1978) taught mildly behaviorally handicapped peers to initiate positive social interactions with three autistic students. As a result the autistic children's social interaction increased. However, social interaction decreased to baseline levels after the intervention was removed. Another study compared the effectiveness of having a mildly handicapped peer initiate social interaction with prompting and reinforcing social play (Strain et al., 1979). Both procedures were effective in increasing positive social behavior.

Almond, Rodgers, and Krug (1979) involved 78 elementary students in tutoring 16 severely handicapped, nonlanguage, autistic students. The elementary students were trained to give directions, help (physically prompt), and reinforce. While this was not an experimental study, six volunteers were randomly selected and their tutoring effectiveness was reported as the percentage of appropriate teaching behavior. The scores ranged from 75 to 100%. In another public school program, teachers trained three nonhandicapped, middle school students to tutor two autistic adolescents (Campbell, Scaturro, & Lickson, 1983). No data were reported but the authors stated that the program was successful and four additional students volunteered to be tutors.

Two experiments have demonstrated the effectiveness of using student tutors with autistic children. Young, West, Clare, Jordan, and Stover (1983) trained six elementary students to conduct therapy sessions with three severely handicapped autistic children. The peer therapists were fourth through sixth grade students. Four of them were considered above average students by their teachers, one was considered an underachiever, and one was learning disabled. The students had no prior training or experience with autistic or handicapped children; however, out of curiosity they had visited and observed in the autism classroom in their school. They all volunteered to participate as student therapists.

The autistic children were four, five, and seven years old. Child 1 had an expressive vocabulary of three words at the beginning of the project, did not respond to other people, and engaged in self-stimulation. Child 2 was nonvocal (but was starting to use some signs), self-abusive, and engaged in self-stimulation. Child 3 had gaze aversion, was echolalic, and engaged in self-stimulatory behavior. All three had been classified as autistic by a team of professionals at a diagnostic center.

The experiment used a multiple probe variation of a multiple-baseline design across individuals. After baseline data were collected the student therapists were trained in pairs to use discrete trial therapy programs. The specific instructional skills taught to the elementary students included: 1) give the "get ready" command (the autistic children had already mastered the "get ready" core management program), 2) socially reinforce getting ready or use "stand-up/sit-down" overcorrection for not getting ready, 3) present the discriminative stimulus to begin a discrete trial, 4) use verbal and physical prompts to assist the child, 5) use appropriate consequences (reinforce correct responding, give negative feedback on errors, and overcorrect misbehavior),

6) pause for three to five seconds at the end of the trial (intertrial interval) and 7) record data. Correct responses by the autistic students were reinforced with tokens which were exchanged on a fixed ratio schedule for edibles or play activities. Tokens were always paired with social reinforcement.

All six peer tutors were successfully trained by the teacher to conduct tutoring sessions. The training consisted of instructions, demonstrations, and prompts which were gradually faded (see Table 1 for training sequence). The elementary students continued to use the instructional skills through the remainder of the school year (approximately four months) and they demonstrated generalized use of the skills across different autistic children, different target behaviors (behaviors never before taught to the autistic children), and different settings (e.g., one-to-one, small group, playground, lunchroom). Two of the peer tutors continued their volunteer work into the next school year without re-training. The autistic children progressed well under the tutelage of the elementary students.

This study was replicated with three behaviorally handicapped elementary students (Young, Jenson, Paoletti, Knoch, Rovner, & Cameron, 1983). The behaviorally handicapped peer tutors were successful at teaching autistic children, and the opportunity to tutor became a reinforcing activity that served to increase their appropriate behavior. Peer tutoring by handicapped and nonhandicapped students is a cost-effective resource available for use in the education of autistic children. It also has side benefits of prompting peer interactions and friendships (see below).

COMMUNITY INTEGRATION OF AUTISTIC CHILDREN

In the past, autistic children have had few opportunities to interact with the nonhandicapped. They have, in fact, been almost totally excluded from public school programs (Lovaas & Koegel, 1973; Lovaas, Schreibman, & Koegel, 1974; Russo & Koegel, 1977). However, litigation and legislation during the 1970s have established that the public education system is responsible for educating the severely handicapped, including autistic children and youth. Since legal actions and social trends have promoted deinstitutionalization and increased community integration, educational services for autistic persons are being provided in regular public schools. Autistic students are coming in contact with nonhandicapped individuals on school buses, at lunch,

TABLE 1
Peer Tutors' Training Sequence

1) Peer tutor and teacher discuss discrete trial components.
2) Peer tutor and teacher role play a therapy session.
   (a) Get ready stimulus and consequation
   (b) Discriminative stimuli presentations
   (c) Parameters of correct responses and subsequent, immediate reinforcement
   (d) Intertrial interval
   (e) Data collection for correct, incorrect, prompted, and irrelevant responses
3) Peer tutor observes teacher conducting a session (five to 20 trials).
4) Peer tutor collects data while teacher conducts session (five to 20 trials), or until 100% reliability is obtained with no prompts from teacher.
5) Peer tutor collects data and positively reinforces the child as appropriate (five to 20 trials), or until 100% proficiency with no prompts from teacher.
   (a) Immediate social reinforcement
   (b) Primary reinforcement
   (c) Secondary reinforcement (accumulation of tokens or points for payoff)
6) Peer tutor conducts session with teacher in the instructional booth, prompting as necessary (20 trials at 80% accuracy of teaching proficiency).
   (a) Presentation of discriminative stimulus (S^Ds)
   (b) Positive or negative consequence of response
   (c) Intertrial interval
   (d) Data collection
   (e) Changing program steps (reduction of prompting and modeling)
7) Peer tutor conducts session with teacher outside of instructional booth, prompting as necessary three consecutive sessions at 90% teaching proficiency.
8) Peer tutor conducts session with no teacher present (weekly observations from teacher and feedback as necessary) (maintain 90% teaching proficiency and 100% reliability with data collection).
9) Peer tutor conducts unique session (new task to be taught and/or different autistic child), teacher prompting as necessary (90% proficiency for 20 trials).

(Young, West, Clare, Jordan, & Stover, 1983)

on playgrounds, and, to some extent, during regular classroom activities (e.g., art, music).

The integration of autistic children does not guarantee social interaction with nonhandicapped students (see Walker, McConnell, and Clarke, this volume). Characteristics such as lack of appropriate speech, social isolation, self-stimulation, and lack of appropriate play (Koegel, Egel, & Dunlap, 1980; Schopler & Bristol, 1980) interfere with the reciprocally reinforcing relationship that normally occurs in social interactions. Stainback and Stainback (1982) recommend the use of peers as change agents to increase social interactions. Young et al., (1983) found that prior to training, peers were frustrated because of the nonresponding or inappropriate response by the autistic children. After they became competent in the use of the instructional skills, the peers enjoyed their interaction with the autistic children. In free play situations, such as recess, they interacted with each other in a normal way; however, the elementary students recognized times when the autistic children were not responding appropriately and prompted and reinforced correct social behavior. On a few occasions they also appropriately used overcorrection procedures for self-stimulation, which resulted in an immediate suppression of the inappropriate behavior. Once the peers were comfortable with the autistic children, interactions occurred throughout the day in many different settings. Community integration, coupled with peer training, has great potential for improving the amount and quality of social interaction with autistic children.

Another benefit of integration is the use of peers as models for autistic children. Egel, Richman, and Koegel (1981) demonstrated that autistic children can learn by observing the behavior of normal peers. The newly learned skills were retained after the peer models were removed from training. Varni et al. (1979) assessed the effects of observational learning on 15 autistic child and adult models. The results were minimal and the authors suggested that stimulus overselectivity may have accounted for the failure to learn. Egel, Richman, and Button (1982) suggested that it may have been due to the fact that they were working with lower functioning autistic children. Another possible reason for the different results in the two studies may be the use of peer versus adult models. Autistic children may respond better to peers.

SUMMARY

While relatively little is known about autism, great strides have been made in treating autistic persons and integrating them into the community. The behavioral treatment approach has been very effective in producing change, but the maintenance and generalization of these changes remains a major challenge. Having parents involved in treatment greatly enhances the maintenance of newly learned behavior and increases the probability that the behavior will generalize to nontraining conditions. Family and peers are becoming major resources for successful intervention, but more research is needed on how they can benefit autistic children. In particular, research is needed on how to maintain improved social interactions and generalize the social behavior to nontraining settings and persons.

The core behavior management programs developed by Jenson et al. (1980) provide a standardized curriculum and instructional approach that can be utilized in a variety of settings by different trainers (professionals, volunteers, parents, siblings, and peers). These programs assist autistic children in acquiring basic learning prerequisites needed to function in educational settings where students are taught in groups. The prerequisite skills also provide a foundation for the acquisition of higher level skills. Comprehensive efforts by service providers and researchers herald a promising future for the treatment, acceptance, and community integration of autistic persons.

REFERENCES

ALMOND, P., RODGERS, S., & KRUG, D. (1979). Mainstreaming: A model for including elementary students in the severely handicapped classroom. *Teaching Exceptional Children, 11,* 135-139.

AMERICAN PSYCHIATRIC ASSOCIATION (1980). *Diagnostic and statistical manual of mental disorders* (3rd ed.). Washington, DC: American Psychiatric Association.

BAILEY, S. L. (1981). Stimulus overselectivity in learning disabled children. *Journal of Applied Behavior Analysis, 14,* 239-248.

BARTAK, L., & RUTTER, M. (1976). Differences between mentally retarded and normally intelligent autistic children. *Journal of Autism and Childhood Schizophrenia, 6,* 109-120.

BARTAK, L., RUTTER, M., & COX, A. (1975). A comparative study of infantile autism and specific developmental receptive language disorder. 1. The children. *British Journal of Psychiatry, 126,* 127-145.

CAMPBELL, A., SCATURRO, J., & LICKSON, J. (1983). Peer tutors help autistic students enter the mainstream. *Teaching Exceptional Children, 15*(2), 64-69.

CARR, E. (1977). The motivation of self-injurious behavior: A review of some hypotheses. *Psychological Bulletin, 84,* 800-816.

CARR, E. G. (1979). Teaching autistic children to use sign language: Some research issues. *Journal of Autism and Developmental Disabilities, 9,* 345-360.

CARR, E. (1982). The motivation of self-injurious behavior. In R. L. Koegel, A. Rincover, & A. L. Egel (Eds.), *Educating and understanding autistic children.* San Diego, CA: College-Hill Press.

CARR, E. G., NEWSOM, C. D., & BINKOFF, J. A. (1976). Stimulus control of self-destructive behavior in a psychotic child. *Journal of Abnormal Child Psychology, 4,* 139-153.

CHESS, S. (1977). Follow-up report on autism in congenital rubella. *Journal of Autism and Childhood Schizophrenia, 7,* 68-81.

COHEN, D. J., CAPARULO, B. K., GOLD, J. R., WALDO, M. C., SHAYWITZ, B. A., RUTTENBURG, B. A., & RIMLAND, B. (1978). Agreement in diagnosis: Clinical assessment and behavior rating scales for pervasively disturbed children. *Journal of the American Academy of Child Psychiatry, 17,* 589-603.

CREAK, M. (1961). Schizophrenic syndrome in childhood. Progress report of the working party. *British Medical Journal, 2,* 889-890.

DEMYER, M. K., BARTON, S., ALPERN, G. D., KIMBERLIN, C., ALLEN, J., YANG, E., & STEELE, R. (1974). The measured intelligence of autistic children. *Journal of Autism and Childhood Schizophrenia, 4,* 42-60.

DEMYER, M. K., BARTON, S., DEMYER, W. E., NORTON, J. A., ALLEN, J., & STEELE, R. (1973). Prognosis in autism: A follow-up study. *Journal of Autism and Childhood Schizophrenia, 3,* 199-246.

DEMYER, M., HINGTGEN, J. N., & JACKSON, R. K. (1981). Infantile autism reviewed: A decade of research. *Schizophrenia Bulletin, 7,* 388-451.

DEVANY, J., & RINCOVER, A. (1982). Self-stimulatory behavior and sensory reinforcement. In R. Koegel, A. Rincover, & A. L. Egel (Eds.), *Educating and understanding autistic children.* San Diego, CA: College-Hill Press.

DONDER, D., & NIETUPSKI, J. (1981). Nonhandicapped adolescents teaching playground skills to their mentally retarded peers: Toward a less restrictive middle school environment. *Education and Training of the Mentally Retarded, 16*(4), 270-276.

DONNELLAN, A., GOSSAGE, L. D., LA VIGNA, G. W., SCHULER, A., & TRAPHAGEN, J. D. (1977). *Teaching makes a difference.* California State Department of Education.

EGEL, A. L. (1982). Programming the generalization and maintenance of treatment gains. In R. L. Koegel, A. Rincover, & A. L. Egel (Eds.), *Educating and understanding autistic children.* San Diego, CA: College-Hill Press.

EGEL, A. L., RICHMAN, G. S., & BUTTON, C. B. (1982). Integration of autistic children with normal children. In R. L. Koegel, A. Rincover, & A. L. Egel (Eds.), *Educating and understanding autistic children.* San Diego, CA: College-Hill Press.

EGEL, A. L., RICHMAN, G. S., & KOEGEL, R. L. (1981). Normal peer models and autistic children's learning. *Journal of Applied Behavior Analysis, 14,* 3-12.

FAVELL, J. E., MCGIMSEY, J. F., & JONES, M. L. (1978). The use of physical restraint in the treatment of self-injury and as a positive reinforcer. *Journal of Applied Behavior Analysis, 11,* 235-241.

FENRICK, N., & MCDONNELL, J. J. (1980). Junior high school students as teachers of the severely retarded: Training and generalization. *Education and Training of the Mentally Retarded, 15*(3), 187-194.

FOLSTEIN, S., & RUTTER, M. (1978). A twin study of individuals with infantile autism. In M. Rutter & E. Schopler (Eds.), *Autism: A reappraisal of concepts and treatment.* New York: Plenum Press.

FOXX, R. M. (1977). Attention training: The use of overcorrection avoidance to increase eye contact of autistic and retarded children. *Journal of Applied Behavior Analysis, 10,* 489-499.

FRANKEL, F., FREEMAN, B. J., RITVO, E., & PARDO, R. (1978). The effect of environmental stimulation upon the stereotyped behavior of autistic children. *Journal of Autism and Childhood Schizophrenia, 8,* 389-394.

FRANKEL, F., & SIMMONS, J. Q. (1976). Self-injurious behavior in schizophrenic and retarded children. *American Journal of Mental Deficiency, 80,* 512-522.

FREEMAN, B. J., & RITVO, E. R. (1976). Parents as paraprofessionals. In E. R. Ritvo (Ed.), *Autism: Diagnosis, current research, and management.* New York: Spectrum Publications.

GLADSTONE, B. W., & SHERMAN, J. A. (1975). Developing generalized behavior modification skills in high school students working with retarded children. *Journal of Applied Behavior Analysis, 8,* 169-180.

HARLOW, H. F., & HARLOW, S. (1971). Psychopathology in monkeys. In H. D. Kimmel (Ed.), *Experimental psychopathology: Recent research and theory.* New York: Academic Press.

HAYDEN, A. H., & MCGINNESS, G. D. (1977). Bases for early intervention. In E. Sontag, J. Smith, & N. Certo (Eds.), *Educational programming for the severely and profoundly handicapped.* Reston, VA: Council for Exceptional Children.

HEWITT, F. M. (1964). Teaching reading to an autistic boy through operant conditioning. *American Journal of Orthopsychiatry, 17,* 613-618.

HILL, J., & WEHMAN, P. (1980). Integration of severely and profoundly handicapped youth into community-level recreation programs: A social validation. In P. Wehman & J. Hill (Eds.), *Instructional programming for severely handicapped youth.* Richmond, VA: School of Education, Virginia Commonwealth University. Reprinted in ERIC System, EC 132 834, 1981.

HUTT, C., & OUNSTED, C. (1970). Gaze aversion and its significance in childhood autism. In S. J. Hutt & C. Hutt (Eds.), *Behavior studies in psychiatry.* New York: Pergamon Press.

ITARD, J. M. (1962). *The wild boy of Aveyron.* New York: Appleton-Century-Crofts.

JENSON, W. R., & REAVIS, K. (1982). *Autism decision matrix.* (Available from) Utah State Board of Education, 250 East Fifth South, Salt Lake City, Utah 84111.

JENSON, W. R., & CBTU STAFF (1980). *Parent training curriculum for families of developmentally disabled children.* (Available from) Salt Lake County Mental Health, 668 South 1300 East, Salt Lake City, Utah 84102.

KANNER, L. (1943). Autistic disturbances of affective contact. *Nervous Child, 2,* 217-250.

KANNER, L. (1971). Follow-up study of 11 autistic children originally reported in 1943. *Journal of Autism and Childhood Schizophrenia, 1,* 119-145. ·

KING, P. D. (1975). Early infantile autism: Relation to schizophrenia. *Journal of the American Academy of Child Psychiatry, 14,* 666-682.

KOEGEL, R. L., & COVERT, A. (1972). The relationship of self-stimulation to learning in autistic children. *Journal of Applied Behavior Analysis, 5,* 381-387.

KOEGEL, R. L., EGEL, A. L., & DUNLAP, G. (1980). Learning characteristics of autistic children. In W. S. Sailor, B. Wilcox, & L. J. Brown (Eds.), *Methods of instruction with severely handicapped students.* Baltimore, MD: Brookes Publishers.

KOEGEL, R. L., FIRESTONE, P. B., KRAMME, K. W., & DUNLAP, G. (1974). Increasing spontaneous play by suppressing self-stimulation in autistic children. *Journal of Applied Behavior Analysis, 7,* 521-528.

KOEGEL, R. L., GLAHN, T. J., & NIEMINEN, G. S. (1978). Generalization of parent-training results. *Journal of Applied Behavior Analysis, 11,* 95-109.

KOEGEL, R. L., RINCOVER, A., & EGEL, A. L. (Eds.). (1982). *Educating and understanding autistic children.* San Diego, CA: College-Hill Press.

KOEGEL, R. L., SCHREIBMAN, L., BRITTEN, K. R., BURKE, J. C., & O'NEILL, R. E. (1982). A comparison of parent training to direct child treatment. In R. L. Koegel, A. Rincover, & A. L. Egel (Eds.), *Educating and understanding autistic children.* San Diego, CA: College-Hill Press.

KRUG, D. A., ARICK, J. R., & ALMOND, P. J. (1979). *Autism screening instrument for educational planning.* Portland, OR: A.S.I.E.P. Publishers.

LOCKYER, L., & RUTTER, M. (1969). A five to fifteen-year follow-up study of infantile psychosis. III. Psychological aspects. *British Journal of Psychiatry, 115,* 865-882.

LOTTER, V. (1978). Follow-up studies. In M. Rutter & E. Schopler (Eds.), *Autism: A reappraisal of concepts and treatment.* New York: Plenum Press.

LOVAAS, O. I. (1966). A program for the establishment of speech in psychotic children. In J. K. Wing (Ed.), *Early childhood autism.* Oxford: Pergamon Press.

LOVAAS, O. I. (1977). *The autistic child: Language development through behavior modification.* New York: Irvington.

LOVAAS, O. I., & BUCHER, B. D. (Eds.). (1974). *Perspectives in behavior modification with deviant children.* Englewood Cliffs, NJ: Prentice Hall.

LOVAAS, O. I., FREITAS, L., NELSON, K., & WHALEN, C. (1967). The establishment of imitation and its use for establishment of complex behavior in schizophrenic children. *Behaviour Research and Therapy, 5,* 171-181.

LOVAAS, O. I., KOEGEL, R. L., & SCHREIBMAN, L. (1979). Stimulus overselectivity in autism: A review of the research. *Psychological Bulletin, 86,* 1236-1254.

LOVAAS, O. I., KOEGEL, R. L., SIMMONS, J. O., & LONG, J. (1973). Some generalization and follow-up measures on autistic children in behavior therapy. *Journal of Applied Behavior Analysis, 6,* 131-165.

LOVAAS, I., SCHAEFFER, B., & SIMMONS, J. Q. (1965). Building social behavior in autistic children by use of electric shock. *Journal of Experimental Research in Personality, 1*, 99-109.

LOVAAS, O. I., SCHREIBMAN, L., & KOEGEL, R. L. (1974). A behavior modification approach to the treatment of autistic children. *Journal of Autism and Childhood Schizophrenia, 4*, 111-129.

LOVAAS, O. I., SCHREIBMAN, L., KOEGEL, R., & REHM, R. (1971). Selective responding by autistic children to multiple sensory input. *Journal of Abnormal Psychology, 77*, 211-222.

MANZANO, J., & PRALONG, W. (1982). An autistic circle of effective simulation. *Journal of Autism and Developmental Disorders, 12*, 93-94.

MARSHALL, G. R. (1966). Toilet training of an autistic 8-year-old through operant conditioning therapy: A case report. *Behaviour Research and Therapy, 4*, 242-245.

NATIONAL SOCIETY FOR AUTISTIC CHILDREN (1978). Definitions of the syndrome of autism. *Journal of Autism and Childhood Schizophrenia, 8*, 162-167.

NORDQUIST, V. M., & WAHLER, R. G. (1973). Naturalistic treatment of an autistic child. *Journal of Applied Behavior Analysis, 6*, 79-87.

PALUSZNY, M. J. (1979). *Autism: A practical guide for parents and professionals.* New York: Syracuse University Press.

PECK, C. H., APOLLONI, T., & COOKE, T. P. (1978). Teaching retarded preschoolers to imitate the free-play behavior of nonretarded classmates: Training and generalized effects. *Journal of Special Education, 12*, 195-207.

RAGLAND, E. U., KERR, M. M., & STRAIN, P. S. (1978). Behavior of withdrawn autistic children: Effects of peer social interactions. *Behavior Modification, 2*, 565-578.

RAVER, S. A., COOKE, T. P., & APOLLONI, T. (1978). Developing nonretarded toddlers as verbal models for retarded classmates. *Child Study Journal, 8*, 1-8.

REISER, D., & BROWN, J. (1964). Patterns of later development of children with infantile psychosis. *Journal of the American Academy of Child Psychiatry, 3*, 650-667.

RICHER, J. M. (1978). The partial noncommunication of culture to autistic children—An application of human ethology. In M. Rutter & E. Schopler (Eds.), *Autism: A reappraisal of concepts and treatment.* New York: Plenum Press.

RICHER, J., & RICHARDS, M. (1975). Reacting to autistic children: The danger of trying too hard. *British Journal of Psychiatry, 1975, 27*, 526-529.

RIMLAND, B. (1978). Savant capabilities of autistic children and their cognitive implications. In G. Serban (Ed.), *Cognitive defects in the development of mental illness.* New York: Brunner/Mazel.

RINCOVER, A. (1981). *How to use sensory extinction.* Lawrence, KS: H & H Enterprises.

ROMANCZYK, R. G., DIAMANT, C., GOREN, E. R., TRUNELL, G., & HARRIS, S. L. (1975). Increasing isolated and social play in several disturbed children: Intervention and post-intervention effectiveness. *Journal of Autism and Childhood Schizophrenia, 5*, 57-70.

RUSSO, D. C., & KOEGEL, R. L. (1977). A method for integrating an autistic child into a normal public school classroom. *Journal of Applied Behavior Analysis, 10*, 579-590.

RUTTER, M. (1970). Autistic children: Infancy to adulthood. *Seminars in Psychiatry, 2*, 435-450.

RUTTER, M. (1974). The development of infantile autism. *Psychological Medicine, 4*, 147-163.

RUTTER, M. (1978a). Diagnosis and definition of childhood autism. *Journal of Autism and Childhood Schizophrenia, 8*, 139-161.

RUTTER, M. (1978b). Language disorder and infantile autism. In M. Rutter & E. Schopler (Eds.), *Autism: A reappraisal of concepts and treatment.* New York: Plenum Press.

RUTTER, M., GREENFIELD, D., & LOCKYER, L. (1967). A five to fifteen year follow-up study of infantile psychosis. II. Social and behavioral outcome. *British Journal of Psychiatry, 113*, 1183-1199.

SCHOPLER, E. (1978). Confusion in the diagnosis of autism. *Journal of Autism and Childhood Schizophrenia, 8,* 137-138.

SCHOPLER, E., & BRISTOL, M. M. (1980). *Autistic children in public school.* ERIC Exceptional Child Education Report. Reston, VA: Council for Exceptional Children.

SCHOPLER, E., & REICHLER, R. J. (1971). Parents as co-therapists in the treatment of psychotic children. *Journal of Autism and Childhood Schizophrenia, 1,* 87-102.

SCHOPLER, E., REICHLER, R. J., DEVILLIS, R. F., & DALY, K. (1980). Toward objective classification of childhood autism: Childhood Autism Rating Scale (CARS). *Journal of Autism and Developmental Disorders, 10,* 91-103.

SCHOVER, L. R., & NEWSOM, C. D. (1976). Overselectivity, developmental level, and overtraining in autistic and normal children. *Journal of Abnormal Child Psychology, 4,* 289-298.

SCHREIBMAN, L., & LOVAAS, O. I. (1973). Overselective response to social stimuli by autistic children. *Journal of Abnormal Child Psychology, 1,* 152-168.

SCHROEDER, S. R., SCHROEDER, C. S., SMITH, B., & DALLDORF, J. (1978). Prevalence of self-injurious behaviors in a large state facility for the retarded: A three year follow-up study. *Journal of Autism and Childhood Schizophrenia, 8,* 261-269.

STAINBACK, W., & STAINBACK, S. (1982). Social interactions between autistic students and their peers. *Behavioral Disorders, 7,* 75-81.

STRAIN, P. S., KERR, M. M., & RAGLAND, E. U. (1979). Effects of peer-mediated social initiations and prompting/reinforcement procedures on the social behavior of autistic children. *Journal of Autism and Developmental Disorders, 9,* 41-54.

VAN WAGENEN, L., JENSON, W. R., WORSHAM, H., & PETERSEN, P. B. (1983). *The use of sign language as a prompt to teach a verbal color discrimination to a developmentally disabled boy.* Manuscript submitted for publication.

VARNI, J. W., LOVAAS, O. I., KOEGEL, R. L., & EVERETT, N. L. (1979). An analysis of observational learning in autistic and normal children. *Journal of Abnormal Child Psychology, 7,* 31-43.

WALKER, G. R., HINERMAN, P. S., JENSON, W. R., & PETERSEN, P. B. (1981). Sign language as a prompt to teach a verbal "Yes" and "No" discrimination to an autistic boy. *Child Behavior Therapy, 3,* 77-87.

WILHELM, H., & LOVAAS, O. I. (1976). Stimulus overselectivity: A common feature in autism and mental retardation. *American Journal of Mental Deficiency, 81,* 227-241.

WING, L., & GOULD, J. (1979). Severe impairments of social interaction and associated abnormalities in children: Epidemiology and classification. *Journal of Autism and Developmental Disorders, 9,* 11-29.

WOLFF, P. H. (1967). The role of biological rhythms in early psychological development. *Bulletin of the Menninger Clinic, 31,* 197-218.

YOUNG, K. R., JENSON, W. R., PAOLETTI, P., KNOCH, E., ROVNER, L., & CAMERON, S. (1983, May). *Teaching behaviorally handicapped students to conduct therapy sessions with autistic children.* Paper presented at the meeting of the Association for Behavior Analysis, Milwaukee, WI.

YOUNG, K. R., WEST, R. P., CLARE, S., JORDAN, J., & STOVER, T. (1983, May). *Training elementary students to conduct therapy sessions with autistic children.* Paper presented at the meeting of the Association for Behavior Analysis, Milwaukee, WI.

9

Prevention of Child Abuse Through the Development of Parent and Child Competencies

DAVID A. WOLFE

Within a brief 15 year timespan, our knowledge and understanding of family violence has evolved from clinical descriptions of the families to well articulated and verifiable theories. The attention of social scientists to the problem of child abuse has had a significant impact on elevating the problem to the status of scientific investigation. It is this juncture between theoretical explanations of the problem and the integration of theory with practice that affords us the privilege of reviewing our direction and questioning our assumptions. In particular, we should be concerned that so little data currently exists on *altering* abusive patterns in the family, as opposed to explaining them. Perhaps the conjured image of violence between parent and child prohibits us from accepting a parsimonious and meaningful explanation of the

Preparation of this chapter was assisted in part by Grant #MA-7807 from the Medical Research Council of Canada, in support of two projects in the study and prevention of child abuse. The author gratefully acknowledges the efforts of members of his research team studying early intervention approaches: Cathy Koverola, Ian Manion, Betty Edwards, and graduate students in clinical and developmental psychology.

events which occur between the two that might lead to abuse. Although efforts at explaining the etiology of child abuse have made important contributions to our understanding, we need also to avoid immobilization that often surrounds such complex and multicausal social problems. Several possibilities for planning early intervention programs can be debated on the basis of current, available information, and the purpose of this chapter is to suggest which directions may be beneficial.

Although the implications are bothersome, the prevention concepts discussed herein are based on the evidence that child abuse, like other forms of intrafamilial violence, is not due to some extremely abnormal or pathological influence. To the contrary, the Family Violence Research Program at the University of New Hampshire has been studying these phenomena among a wide sample of American families since 1970, and they conclude:

> While granting that some instances of intrafamily violence are an outgrowth of social or psychological pathology, we maintain that physical violence between family members is a normal part of family life in most societies, and in American society in particular. (Gelles & Straus, 1979, p. 549)

The alternative to viewing child abuse as an extremely abnormal behavior is to view the abusive act as the culmination of numerous, interrelated events in the family. Attempts to unravel the critical problems in the family which are likely to provoke aggression have resulted in the discovery of more similarities than differences among abusive families and other distressed, but non-abusive, families (Wolfe, in press). It is these important realizations that direct us more toward a stance of family assistance and support, rather than ostracism and punishment.

To argue that child abuse is not abnormal is not to imply that it is normal, common, or tolerable. In a manner of speaking, abuse exists because we allow the known and suspected causes to flourish unhampered in the family and community systems until we are forced to protect the child. This is a grossly ineffective and hazardous approach which is still very commonly employed. The alternative to the child protection approach will involve radical changes in our current system of services to families. However, this chapter will focus upon research findings which support the premise that a large percentage of abusive incidents may be prevented (Standing Senate Committee on Health, Welfare, & Science, 1980). Furthermore, the changes necessary for retooling from a protection to a prevention model may be less complex and more feasible than many of our current theories suggest.

THEORETICAL INTEGRATION AND SHORTCOMINGS

Gelles and Straus (1979) report on 15 theories which address the known data on child abuse. The number of theories does not seem surprising when one considers that this problem has received considerable public attention and funding, and a great deal of research effort has been directed towards etiology (Alvy, 1975). According to these authors, the two distinctive key elements of these theories are the social learning interactional processes among family members and the frustration-aggression relationship. Taken together, these two theoretical dimensions provide ample coverage of the known information on child abuse as well as other forms of violence. Neither component is static or assumed to be inherent in the individual or family—social learning and aggression processes are represented as an ongoing, reciprocal function of the intra- and extra-family events which contribute to the likelihood of family violence. These processes will be reviewed briefly before presenting findings which challenge some of the overgeneralizations which have sprung from these theories.

The social learning or social interactional model of child abuse places heavy emphasis on the escalation of coercion and aversive interactions among family members, which may culminate in physical injury to the weakest family member. Both parent and child are believed to contribute to the coercive interchanges, and the critical factors which are assumed to differentiate abusive families from non-abusive are primarily environmental (e.g., levels of stress and support), individual (e.g., childrearing skills, child difficulty, coping ability), and consequential (e.g., short-term reduction of aversiveness following punishment). The occurrence of physical punishment and the many "essential ingredients" of the abusive family are well incorporated into this interactional model of abuse. Further definition of this model is presented by Friedman, Sandler, Hernandez, and Wolfe (1981), Parke and Collmer (1975), and Patterson (1982).

In addition to the social learning components of abuse, Vasta (1982) stresses the critical importance of what he and Knutson (1978) have termed "irritable aggression." To complete the theoretical abuse scenario, physical punishment (via social learning) explodes into physical injury and abuse due to the perpetrator's level of emotional arousal.

Such arousal may be linked, historically, to the abuser's learned "hyper-reactivity" or helplessness/frustration when faced with aversive events, a process that is not well understood but certainly worthy of careful investigation. Citing studies that link both physiological and cognitive arousal to acts of human aggression, Vasta (1982) has provided another critical link in our explanation of why one parent might abuse while another does not.

The above conceptualizations of child abuse together provide a very comprehensive explanation of abuse which has received initial empirical support (Vasta & Copitch, 1981) and has led to important treatment gains (Isaacs, 1982). However, several comparisons of abusive and control families have led to equivocal findings which challenge the implication that abusive families are significantly different from other families on social, behavioral, or related theoretical factors. In a carefully designed study to identify social, parental, or child variables that differentiate abusers from non-abusers, Starr (1982) reported that very few meaningful differences emerged when abusive and control groups were carefully matched. The author acknowledged that abusive mothers "are generally functioning less adequately" than other mothers, but both groups appeared to have considerable overlap rather than basic differences. Similarly, in a large multivariate study of the factors which differentiate abusers from non-abusers, Gaines, Sandgrund, Green, and Power (1978) could account for only 12% of the variance among abusing, neglecting, and normal mothers using 12 variables of theoretical importance. The authors concluded that factors related to "general levels of family stress" contributed more to maltreatment than any personality variable related to the parent or child. Bolton, Laner, and Kane (1980) reported from their sample of 4,851 child abuse cases in Arizona that more than one-third involved a mother who was an adolescent at the birth of one of her children; however, Kinard and Klerman (1980) presented findings that the hypothesized link between teenage parenting and child abuse disappeared when socioeconomic factors were controlled in their sample. These representative studies, therefore, remind us that factors associated with child abuse are often extremely complex and do not reliably distinguish abusive and non-abusive families (Wolfe, in press).

Similar concerns about meaningful differences between abusers and non-abusers emerge from the data on the behavioral and emotional patterns of the abused child. Contrary to expectations, the first two controlled studies of abused children reported that these children do not show significantly abnormal developmental behaviors when compared to carefully matched controls. In a follow-up study of abused children in which matched controls were employed, Elmer (1977) concluded that the effects on child development of lower-class membership may be as powerful as abuse. In their large-scale home observational study of abusive and comparison families, Burgess and Conger (1978) also concluded that although abused children displayed high rates of negative behavior, they did not appear to behave in a fashion remarkably different from controls. Wolfe and Mosk (1983) investigated the behavior exhibited by abused children in comparison to a matched sample of non-abused children from distressed families who were involved with a child welfare agency. This comparison revealed that the negative psychological consequences of abuse could not be distinguished from the consequences of severe family distress on the basis of the measures of child social competence and behavior problems. The investigators concluded from these findings that the influences of pervasive family problems may be as dramatic as physical violence in contributing to child behavioral disturbance. In a recent review of the developmental effects of child abuse, Toro (1982) summarized the major studies on the abused child and stated that on the basis of current data we cannot conclude that abused children are measurably different from other children who have been matched on critical family factors.

These findings on the characteristics of the abusive parent and the abused child point to a major concern: When levels of stress and family environmental factors are carefully controlled, the theoretical differences between abusive and non-abusive families begin to fade. Moreover, few data on father-child interaction in abusive families have been reported. Thus the findings to date are incomplete insofar as differences between abusive mothers and fathers may contribute to our understanding. What emerges from the comparative studies of abusive and non-abusive families are not two distinct family patterns related to etiological factors of child abuse; instead, several distinct responses emerge which parents may emit when faced with any one of a number of stressful circumstances, such as physical aggression towards the child, withdrawal from caring for the child, increases in maladaptive coping, or increases in effective coping. Although we do not know what "causes" these different parental responses, the inference has been upon a parental defect which renders some parents incapable of controlling their behavior. Conversely, it is plausible to assume that many parents simply do not know how to initiate or maintain consistent, non-aversive interactions with their child, and need very early assistance and education. At this point in time we must accept that our understanding of why some parents respond differently to stressful circumstances is severely limited. Rather than imposing a pathological explanation of child abuse in the absence of clear data, it may be more advantageous for intervention purposes to consider what these families are doing that may lead to violence and to emphasize methods for strengthening their coping abilities. This approach would appear reasonable, given our current extremely limited ability to eradicate the large number of suspected contributing causes of abuse.

COMPETENCE MODEL VERSUS DEFECT MODEL OF ABUSE

Since child abuse appears to occur only in a relatively small proportion of the families who share many of the high-risk characteristics, it seems imperative that we focus more attention on the abilities which some of these parents have or could develop. For purposes of prevention and early intervention, as opposed to theory construction and validation, it may prove more beneficial to develop competency and support for the parents considered to be "high-risk" than to locate and treat the elusive "defect" in parents found to be abusive. We need to consider the long-range benefits of recognizing "high-risk" family characteristics and offering assistance in modifying those problematic elements which are amenable to change.

White (1959) argued that competence is a motivational concept which explains the process of learning to interact effectively with the environment. Over the last decade community psychologists developed a practical model of ways in which stressed individuals learn to cope with adversity and to develop competence. This model focuses on enhancing an individual's functioning by improving the skills needed to cope with environmental stressors (Holahan & Spearly, 1980), and places emphasis on the critical health factors that may be boosted to counteract adversity. Applying this principle to abusive families, Helfer (1982, p. 253) states: "This decision is to determine whether or not the ultimate purpose [of intervention] is to prevent something harmful; i.e., abuse and/or neglect to a child, or to enhance something positive; i.e., an improved interaction between a parent and a child."

A prevention-oriented approach to child abuse, therefore, must propose methods to alter the major high-risk factors associated with current theoretical models of abuse by planning strategies for promoting competence of the parents and children. The overriding assumption in this model is that abuse is learned behavior that can be conceptualized in both instrumental and respondent terms (Vasta, 1982), and as such may be prevented if appropriate learning opportunities are available. The goals and rationale for such a program include: 1) the development of strong positive habits of childrearing through successful and non-aversive parent-child interactions at an early stage; 2) improvement in the parent's abilities to cope with stress through exposure to a mental health support system; and 3) the development of the child's adaptive behaviors which will contribute to the child's emotional and psychological adjustment.

The following target areas for the prevention of abuse are conceptualized on the basis of the need for feasible alternatives to treating abusive families *ex post facto*. By reviewing several of the major characteristics of the abuser and the child, proposals will emphasize ways in which these target groups may be reached at an earlier point in time. The concepts discussed will be limited to parent and child deficits which often emerge during postnatal and early childhood periods and which could benefit from educational and training procedures currently available. Emphasis will be placed on the interactional behaviors exhibited among family members rather than upon extra-familial events (e.g., social isolation, unemployment), although these are certainly important additional areas of prevention for study.

MODIFYING PARENTAL RISK FACTORS

Despite the number of contributing factors and individual differences, researchers have been able to agree on certain areas of parental behavioral and psychological functioning which appear to be critical in determining the likelihood of abusive behavior. The following sections will discuss several of the major psychological and behavioral deficiencies that have been highlighted in the child abuse literature for the purpose of clarifying intervention and prevention objectives.

Cognitive and Psychological Abilities of the Parent

Abusive parents have been described as lacking a proper understanding of their child's developmental abilities, displaying a negative or self-centered attitude toward family members, and generally lacking insight into the effects of their behavior upon their children. Authors have speculated that these attitudinal and motivational liabilities of the parent are closely related to the parent's own childhood experiences and adulthood adjustment (Spinetta & Rigler, 1972). The difficulty of altering or defining these pervasive interpersonal behavior patterns poses a substantial burden on mental health services (Alvy, 1975). Alternatively, we may focus on more specific aspects of the parent-child relationship and place less emphasis on the parent's intrinsic adaptation. At this point in time it may be especially important to assist families in those areas that are both problematic and modifiable and to be willing to accept a rate of progress that is measured in relative terms. Attitudinal and personality variables which interfere with effective coping responses merit special concern for establishing reasonable and attainable goals for these families.

The theoretical emphasis upon the abuser's distinctive personality characteristics has received little direct support (Alvy, 1975; Spinetta & Rigler, 1972), yet some meaningful information emerges when certain parental characteristics are more adequately defined and measured. For example, Brunnquell, Crichton, and Egeland (1981) view parental personality and attitudinal variables as important indicators of the parent's integrative functioning, rather than explanations or predictors of abuse. These authors approached the issue of psychological functioning of the parent by dividing their sample of 267 "high-risk" mother-infant pairs into high and low subgroups that could be reliably distinguished on several measures of maternal care and interest. This methodology was employed to determine whether important parental characteristics were associated with abuse and neglect by the time the child was three months old. While they found no set of parental abilities or attitudes to be clearly associated with abuse and neglect, they did find that certain maternal characteristics were related to quality of caretaking. Mothers in the Excellent Care group were found to be of higher intelligence, reacted positively to pregnancy, and had more positive expectations and a better understanding concerning their parental role than parents in the Inadequate Care group. The authors tie these findings to the importance of early intervention by stating:

> It appears that the mother at risk for abuse or neglect is characterized during pregnancy by a lack of understanding and knowledge concerning parent-child relationships and a negative reaction to pregnancy. After the baby arrives, her anxiety and fear increase in response to the difficulty presented by the baby. She is unable to understand the ambivalence she experiences and responds to her anxiety and fear by becoming more hostile and

suspicious. Her increased hostility and suspiciousness interfere further with her ability to relate to the baby and cope with the demands of the situation. (p. 689)

The complexities of parental attitudinal characteristics are enormous, and several authors have raised concerns about their value in a prevention approach to child abuse due to lack of clarity and resistance to change (Alvy, 1975; Burgess & Richardson, 1984). The relationship between attitudes and behavior in disturbed parent-child relationships has not been well-supported, unless the specific domain of attitudes being studied is clearly relevant to the behavior being observed (Tulkin & Cohler, 1973). The results of the study by Brunnquell et al. (1981) appear to be the only available empirical data which help to clarify this attitude-behavior relationship in a manner that has relevance to child abuse prevention. The parent who is well-prepared for the life changes associated with childrearing is less likely to succumb to the increasing stress factors which prevail. This viewpoint is very congruent with the principles of preventive mental health: Skills, knowledge, and experiences which boost the individual's coping abilities will increase their resistance to the forces which oppose their healthy adjustment (Dohrenwend, 1978). Although we must recognize that a small percentage of abusive and high-risk parents have personality difficulties which may be unresponsive to available intervention approaches, we must also recognize that the majority of these parents is capable of benefiting from non-intrusive methods of helping them to cope more effectively with life changes. By setting our goals in close accordance with the parent's cognitive and psychological abilities, we may increase the impact of our early intervention efforts while avoiding the difficulty of prolonged involvement.

In order to maximize a parent's childrearing competence, we must consider more carefully the benefits of approaches to assist them in. understanding and accepting the demands of their role. Several authors have reported on the use of therapeutic approaches with abusive parents, although very limited treatment outcome data are available to evaluate their effectiveness or value. For example, Pollock and Steele (1972) emphasized the importance of supportive counseling for parents which provides the parents with assistance in dealing with crises and helps them to develop stronger coping skills through individual therapy. Ambrose, Hazzard, and Haworth (1980) reported on their development of a group therapy approach for abusive parents which stresses cognitive-behavioral techniques for dealing with feelings of depression, anxiety, and anger. In discussing their findings with high-risk parents, Brunnquell et al. (1981) emphasized an intervention approach which focuses on integration of the mother's reactions, feelings, and perceptions of day-to-day tasks with her infant, which requires a concerned worker who is interested in the individual needs of the client. Clearly, a prevention program must take into consideration the importance of one-to-one counseling and education with the parent, preferably during pregnancy or early infancy. Such a prevention component is certainly within the capabilities of our current child welfare system, provided that a re-emphasis upon early education and assistance is forthcoming. We will also see, in the next section, that efforts to assist parents in their childrearing *abilities* may have a significant and valuable influence on parental attitudes and expectations as well.

Behavioral Abilities of the Parent

In addition to attitudinal and personality factors which impair effective parenting, abusive parents have commonly been described as ineffective, inadequate, verbally and physically negative towards their child, and generally lacking in a behavioral repertoire that is necessary for childrearing responsibilities. For example, Ainsworth (1980) and others (Egeland & Vaughn, 1981) have suggested that a "mismatch" between parent and infant may develop at a very early point in the relationship, based primarily on aversive interactions between the two. Once the parent fails to establish an effective interactional style with the infant or young child, continuation and escalation of conflict are more likely to occur. Because these parents have often been raised in punitive environments themselves, they may have never learned appropriate methods for managing their infant's or child's behavior. Although few reliable differences have been found on personality variables when compared with matched controls, interactions among abusive parents and their children have been shown to be aversive and self-defeating (Burgess & Conger, 1978; Reid, Taplin, & Lorber, 1981; Wolfe, Sandler, & Kaufman, 1981), and modification of these patterns may reduce the risk of physical abuse. The following discussion will focus primarily on recent data which suggest at what point our intervention efforts may best benefit the parent-child relationship, and what skills should be included in such a program.

Experiences with the infant and toddler. Several developmental researchers have addressed the concern that child abuse may be related to problems in early attachment between the mother and child. Infant-caregiver attachment develops over time through interactional processes that may have a significant effect upon the quality of later patterns of care (Ainsworth, Blehar, Waters, & Wall, 1978). In a prospective study, Egeland and Sroufe (1981) assessed the differences in attachment among the children of their Excellent Care and Inadequate Care groups and found that the Excellent Care group had a larger percentage of securely attached infants at both 12 and 18 months. Children who had been victims of abuse or neglect were found to reveal significantly more anxious patterns of attachment than others in the sample, which the authors note is often associated with avoidant behavior patterns resulting from chronic unavailability and/or rejection. The abused child was more likely to show patterns of declining functioning over the first two years of life (Egeland & Sroufe, 1981), which these authors attributed to the parents' childrearing deficiencies, rather than to the developmental status of the infant (e.g., prematurity, delivery complications, infant illness, or other factors which might disrupt the initial infant-mother contact). After careful study of the relationship between early parent-infant contact and abuse, these researchers have suggested that whereas mother's personality characteristics, life stress, family circumstances, and baby characteristics are all important factors in our understanding of abuse and neglect, the early relationship between the caregiver and the infant is critical.

Developmental researchers have shown considerable interest in the similarities between abused infants and maternally deprived infants, suspecting that developmental delay of abused children may be a function of parental inadequacy as opposed to physical abuse alone. Dietrich, Starr, and Kaplan (1980) examined the interactive quality of abusive mothers with their infants and found that in addition to engaging in less quantity and variety of stimulation, the abusive mothers were less involved and more passive with their infants than control mothers. Their patterns of interaction were markedly different in terms of physical intimacy, speech, and similar measures of maternal stimulation and involvement. However, the authors noted that the abusive mothers were not grossly inadequate in their parenting abilities, but rather deficient as a group in their methods of caring for the infant. These findings help us to understand the commonly reported observation that abusive parents with young children appear less interested, less capable, and less involved with their child than normal parents. More importantly, the findings lead more directly and specifically to early intervention objectives. Information on the important qualitative aspects of the early parent-child relationship and the developmental level of the child has significantly advanced our thinking, and we can now begin to formulate specific plans for educating and assisting high-risk parents during the most advantageous time periods.

Preliminary evidence supports the feasibility of reducing abuse and neglect through an early focus on the parent-infant relationship. Egeland and Vaughn (1981) reported that one-third of the mothers in their Adequate Care group participated voluntarily in a program which provided extensive parental education and rooming-in periods to enable parents to touch and interact with their newborn. The authors felt such activities may have accounted for differences in adequacy of care over the first year. Similarly, Egeland and Sroufe (1981) found a sizeable percentage of infants in their sample who changed toward secure attachment between 12 and 18 months. Even though the study was not designed specifically to investigate the effects of intervention, Egeland and Sroufe report that involvement of extended family members or major circumstantial changes were significantly related to positive outcomes. Stabilizing influences in the lives of the mother and infant appear to have the expected, desired effect on the infant's development of secured attachment and prosocial behavior, although direct evidence for this conclusion is not yet available for abused and neglected infants.

Epstein (1980) cites a large body of research in child development which underscores the importance of maternal behavior in helping children to overcome developmental difficulties resulting from social and environmental hardships. Her conclusions point to specific qualities of the parent's behavior which will enhance the parent-child relationship and, consequently, reduce the risk of maltreatment. The dimensions include: 1) verbal communication, which provides information to the infant and intellectual stimulation; 2) physical freedom to explore, which allows the infant to develop sensory and motor abilities without undue restriction or control; 3) responsiveness to the infant's needs in a manner that is consistent with his or her developmental level; and 4) positive affect which accompanies all supportive verbal and physical interactions. These four substantive dimensions of parent-infant development are comprised of specific behaviors that are commonly deficient in the inexperienced or inadequate parent. It seems reasonable that such deficiencies could be remediated by helping parents to learn basic activities and necessary behaviors for interacting with their child. Rather than assuming that such parents are *incapable* or *resistant* to learning about their parenting role, an early intervention approach may provide the parents with new behaviors and insights which are congruent with their emotional and intellectual abilities.

The procedures for teaching basic childrearing skills to high-risk parents do not need to be difficult or complex. Recent findings in the field of child development point to critical parental behaviors which can increase the positive strength of the parent-child relationship. For example, a contingent or predictable social environment in the infant's early months is inversely related to the emergence of infant crying in later months (Wahler & Dumas, in press). Ainsworth's (1980) concept of the "insecurely attached" infant is highly congruent with the behavioral data indicating that when the parent responds in an unaffectionate, noncontingent manner to the infant's bids for attention, the aversiveness (i.e., "insecurity") of infant behavior increases over time. Thus, as Wahler and Dumas (in press) have outlined, a mother who is unable to respond contingently to her infant's attentional demands is setting the stage for increasing coercive-avoidance behaviors on the part of the child which will, over time, come to resemble the behavior of the principal caretaker in terms of behavior style. Although we cannot state *why* such parents respond in the manner that they do, it is evident that this strategy is self-defeating. Wahler and Dumas stress the importance of coercive setting events (e.g., stressful daily experiences, aversive situations) which may covary with the mother's lack of contingent and appropriate affection toward the infant. Such events offer a more tangible explanation for changes in parental behavior than those which state that the parent is insensitive due to emotional and personality factors. From a clinical viewpoint, our knowledge of parent-child behavior warrants the development of teaching strategies for parents which apply established learning principles to problems of insufficient and incontingent interactions between high-risk young parents and their small children.

Managing child-related stress. A basic assumption in the social learning model of abuse is that parents have not had exposure to proper parental models or the opportunity to learn more effective child management skills and, therefore, they rely heavily upon punitive or inappropriate responses to the child's behavior. This aspect of the coercive process stresses the interactional nature between the parent and the child, although the parent is often seen as the target for intervention since the aversiveness of the child behavior has been linked to parental contingencies (Patterson, 1982; Wahler & Dumas, in press). In their attempts to maintain control over their child's behavior, a parent may evidence heightened arousal which in turn acts upon the intended degree of physical punishment to turn it into physical violence (Vasta, 1982). Thus, the combination of ineffective child management abilities and physiological arousal can precipitate an abusive episode, especially in the presence of facilitative environmental circumstances (e.g., social isolation, prolonged stress, limited resources).

One reason that physiological responsiveness may be an important variable related to child abuse involves the role of emotional arousal in producing aggressive behavior. Rule and Nesdale (1976) reported that an individual's heightened level of general emotional arousal will facilitate the expression of aggressive acts in the presence of aggressive cues. According to some theories of aggression (Bandura, 1973; Berkowitz, 1974), an aversive child behavior (such as crying or noncompliance) can function as a cue capable of eliciting aggressive parental actions *if* the parent's emotional arousal is sufficiently high. Anecdotal reports from abusive parents suggest this is often the case; these parents frequently indicate they become extremely angry and tense to the point of discomfort when the child exhibits some action the parent finds unpleasant. While physiological and affective arousal can lead to responses other than aggression, the relationship between parental arousal and abusive behavior is one that merits close attention.

Frodi and Lamb (1980) present data which suggest that abusive mothers report more aversion to infant cries than nonabusers, and physiological changes in abusive mothers indicated increased arousal both to infant cries *and* smiles, whereas control mothers responded with arousal only to infant cries. The authors interpret these findings as an indication that abusers may respond to any social elicitation by the infant (crying or smiling) with emotional arousal indicative of displeasure or aversion. Such arousal may serve to facilitate aggressive reactions to child behaviors which are perceived by the parent as unpleasant or undesirable. Wolfe, Fairbank, Kelly, and Bradlyn (1983) reported that physiological response patterns obtained from abusive mothers indicated that videotaped parent-child interactions rated as stressful produced greater arousal than interactions rated as nonstressful. In contrast, matched non-abusive mothers responded to both types of scenes with significantly less physiological arousal.

The findings relating aversive child behavior to parental arousal strongly suggest that high-risk parents will require assistance in monitoring and controlling their hyperreactivity to child-related stress. Thus, methods of assessing and treating high-risk parents' responses to their child and their ability to control arousal are viewed as highly related phenomena which must receive careful attention in a preventative orientation.

Behavioral treatment programs for abusive parents have primarily focused on deficient child management skills implicated in abuse. A recent review by Isaacs (1982) indicated that progress in this area has been generally favorable, based on 11 behavioral treatment studies that have presented outcome data. In our work with these families, we have been pleased by the changes that many parents and children demonstrated following intensive behavioral parent training (e.g., Wolfe & Sandler, 1981; Wolfe et al., 1981; Wolfe, St. Lawrence, Graves, Brehony, Bradlyn, & Kelly, 1982). However, in order to have a significant impact upon the problem of child abuse, we must investigate whether these treatment methods will *prevent* such problems well in advance of their occurrence. It is our impression that behavioral methods offer considerable promise for reducing the coercive process described above, and attention to conditioned arousal (hyperreactivity) at an early stage in the parent-child relationship will considerably advance prevention efforts.

Supported by the seminal work of Patterson (1982) and Wahler (1980) we have recently begun to develop an approach to assisting parents to cope with stress and arousal that includes two intervention components. First, during child management and stimulation training, the parent is taught in vivo desensitization with the child present (following brief preparatory instructions and rehearsal). This allows the parent the opportunity to practice relaxation, diversion, and similar appropriate coping responses in the presence of realistic child cues (such as noncompliance, screaming, and high activity level), with the assistance and feedback of covert therapist prompts using a bug-in-the-ear device. Such rehearsal continues throughout parent training in order to strengthen the parent's behavioral repertoire and to reduce competing and inappropriate reactions to undesirable child behaviors. Second, a staff member works individually with the parent in the home to monitor and deal with daily problems that might interfere with the parent's efforts to control the child non-forcefully. For example, many of our parents are faced with high levels of economic, housing, transportation, and relationship "crises" that accumulate over short time periods and reduce their parenting effectiveness. A staff member who has been trained to problem-solve with the parent can be a valuable source of support to the parent, as well as an integral part of competence enhancement training.

In sum, parental high-risk factors can be conceptualized in terms of the parent's early expectations, interactions, and responses to the infant and young child, as well as his or her capacity to handle child-related stress. Although abusive parents are often described as considerably deficient in these areas, the development of maladaptive childrearing patterns may be prevented through planned educational and experiential activities. This emphasis is directed toward what the parent *does or does not do,* rather than their inherent limitations or personality patterns. Except for the small minority of parents who are severely limited in their interest and ability to care for their infant, attempts to improve the parent's current skills and resources offer a viable approach to child abuse prevention.

MODIFYING CHILD RISK FACTORS

There is considerable evidence that infant and child characteristics can affect the probability of abuse. The "at-risk" status of an infant may be due to mental, physical, or behavioral abnormalities present from birth, or may be due to learned behaviors that increase the likelihood of abuse (Frodi, 1981). At present we cannot determine whether such atypical behavior patterns precipitate abuse or result from abuse (Friedman et al., 1981; Toro, 1982). However, we can aim our early intervention efforts at maladaptive or deficient developmental patterns being displayed by the child in order to foster positive parent/child interactions and child development.

Aversive and Excessive Child Behaviors

The contributions of infant temperament and irritable child behavior toward parental aggression and abuse have been well-documented. Reviews of studies investigating child effects on adults have uncovered several major and distinct problematic behavior patterns of young children which could elicit negative parental responses (Atwater & Morris, 1979; Bell & Harper, 1977). For example, research by Stevens-Long (1973) indicated that a child's activity level may affect the parent's reactions and disciplinary responses by cuing the adult to increase punishment intensity. Similarly, Patterson (1982) reports that aggressive and disruptive children are at-risk for increased punitive reactions from their parents, and whereas many young children exhibit high rates of aggressive behavior, children who later are labeled "socially deviant" are often those whose family members have contributed to the escalation of coercive exchanges. Often such difficult children may be identified at an early developmental age, and it is reasonable to presume that prevention of punitive escalation as well as child deviancy must occur long before the patterns have strongly developed.

As previously discussed, the influence of infant expression upon adult behavior has also received careful investigation in relation to child abuse. Through a process of conditioning, Frodi (1981) has explained that the abusive adult may begin to perceive the infant/toddler as very aversive, even after the aversive features have been outgrown. Thus, aversive characteristics of some infants may place them at particular risk of abuse during early childhood. Since an infant's cry serves an important caregiving function, it is imperative that the unique developmental features that may accompany aversive infant behavior (e.g., prematurity, delayed development, physical or mental handicaps) receive careful assessment and professional attention.

Behavioral Deficits of the Child

It has not been determined whether physical abuse, per se, is actually the most critical variable interfering with normal child development, since factors associated with physical abuse, such as emotional abuse and neglect and socioeconomic factors, may be more critical determinants of child development (Elmer, 1977; Toro, 1982). Issues of causality aside, we must consider the data which indicate that children from abusive environments are, on the average, farther behind in many critical areas of development, which places them in jeopardy of further abuse, school failure, and long-term adjustment problems (Standing Senate Committee on Health, Welfare, & Science, 1980).

In a study of 30 abused and 30 non-abused infants, Appelbaum (1977) found significant differences in the developmental functioning of abused children as early as four months of age on several measures of cognitive and psychomotor development. The author interpreted these findings as indications that inadequate parenting behavior is a more plausible explanation for early delays than actual physical trauma or general environmental deprivation. The data of Egeland and Sroufe (1981) also support the contention that quality of parenting is the major factor involved in develomental delay, stating that, as a group, abused children in their sample appeared relatively retarded by 24 months of age. Thus, certain children may be at-risk as a result of their birth status (e.g., retardation, prematurity), and many other children may begin to show early signs of developmental problems as a consequence of parental inadequacy. Reversing these delays is a high priority for an early intervention program, since such efforts may result in prevention of parental abuse as well as severe developmental handicaps.

Specific areas of functioning that appear to be most relevant to the prevention of abuse include the development of verbal and social abilities. Although a large proportion of children with delayed speech and language development at three years may catch up, such delays may in turn lead to delays in other critical areas (Pawlby & Hall, 1980). Hess and Shipman (cited in Pawlby & Hall, 1980) found that the "teaching style" of lower class mothers is far less explicit and less effective than middle-class mothers, which may in turn affect the child's overall cognitive functioning. An overly restricted linguistic environment might limit the child's opportunity for learning complex language skills and, in turn, result in diminished attention from adults (Atwater & Morris, 1979). A similar reciprocal pattern of adult-child interaction which limits child development has been found in the development of the child's social skills. Experimental studies relating unresponsive child behavior to adult reactions have found that such children receive less attention, help, and praise from adults and were rated less favorably by adults after the interaction (Cantor & Gelfand, cited in Atwater & Morris, 1979). Children with social deficits are more likely to come from disadvantaged and distressed families, and such behavioral deficits seem to perpetuate social rejection and inattention from others (Strain & Shores, 1977).

The implications of these initial findings on the developmental deficits and excesses of abused children are straightforward: Favorable adult responses are associated with positive child behavior. These child behaviors include, at a minimum, expressions of positive affect, moderate activity level, responsiveness to adult instructions and feedback, and age-appropriate language and social skills (Atwater & Morris, 1979). These findings suggest that early intervention efforts should include strategies to enhance the developmental and adaptive abilities of the child, in addition to the adaptive skills and knowledge of the parent.

Unfortunately, very few intervention programs for abuse and neglect have been evaluated which focus on the child's needs at a very early point in time (Helfer, 1982). This is especially troublesome since reviews of studies with non-abused, delayed children have concluded that early intervention can have a sustained and significant impact on the child's cognitive and social development (Carew, 1979). For example,

Belsky, Goode, and Most (1980) investigated the hypothesis that maternal stimulation can foster infant exploratory competence. The mother's behavior was influenced by minimally intrusive visits to the home in which feedback and suggestions were provided to the parent, and in return the child's exploratory abilities were significantly enhanced. A particular strength of this approach was its encouragement of parental abilities and competence instead of inadequacies. The authors suggest that such a supportive strategy develops trust so that more directive methods can be continued with the parents. Comprehensive child abuse early intervention programs can profit greatly from the procedures being investigated by developmental researchers and practitioners with related child populations.

The prevention of child abuse and its long-term consequences, therefore, should be at least a twofold process involving the strengthening of parental competence and pleasurable experiences with their child, as well as the enhancement of the child's adaptive abilities. This conclusion has formed the basis for our current early intervention program with at-risk parents and children. This longitudinal study is aimed at investigating the preventative benefits of early intervention with parents who have insufficient and inappropriate childrearing abilities (Wolfe, 1983). We are applying many of the methods explored in previous studies with abusive and non-abusive parents to a population of parents who are at-risk of abuse, and attempting to improve the overall quality of the parent/child relationship at an early point in time. Although behavioral intervention for abusive parents has produced initially promising findings, modifying parent/child interaction patterns that have been in operation for several years is a difficult and costly task. The current program incorporates several new training methods into child abuse treatment to direct greater emphasis on qualitative aspects of the parent-child relationship, developmentally appropriate activities and skill-rehearsal tasks, and enhancement of adaptive functioning in the child.

CONCLUSIONS

This chapter has reviewed several areas of parental and child functioning which can be operationally applied to child abuse prevention. Since few therapeutically relevant variables have been found when comparing abusive and matched non-abusive parents, the emphasis has been mainly upon a combination of behavioral deficits which may develop into abuse if left unchecked. This viewpoint necessitates a different perspective and approach to assisting abusive families than is currently popular. Unfortunately, the contributions of psychology, psychiatry, and social work toward preventing abuse or treating abusers have focused primarily on pathology, and have led to a disappointingly low impact on the overall problem. Alternatively, many authors have called for a multidisciplinary preventative approach which attacks the problem at all levels (e.g., Belsky, 1980; Cohn, 1982; Helfer, 1982). The contributions which psychology can make toward this effort are extremely tangible and significant.

The psychologist's role in preventing abuse entails methods for enhancing parental competence through education and training. This review has pinpointed several critical areas of need for the parent and child which appear to be amenable to early intervention. First, the parents' skills in teaching new behaviors and handling difficult child behavior can be enhanced through well-documented parent training procedures, involving direct observation, feedback, demonstration, and rehearsal of important skills. Second, a parent who experiences high levels of anxiety, tension, or arousal, and/or who has a child who displays highly aversive behavior, can be taught effective coping strategies such as relaxation and stress management (Denicola & Sandler, 1980). Third, the parents' early experiences and responses to the infant and young child can be enhanced by preparing the young parent for childrearing responsibilities and life changes. This latter goal could be combined with the recognized need for supportive educational guidance and support systems during pre- and post-natal periods. Throughout each of these goals is an implicit emphasis upon enhancement of the child's physical, psychological, and behavioral development. During parent training or supportive counseling, the parent can be taught methods for stimulating the child's language and social development through enjoyable home activities and parent-infant experiences.

During the development of competency-based child abuse prevention programs, other factors which may contribute to success will require consideration. Since we cannot accurately predict who may become abusive, screening parents for involvement in early intervention requires collaboration among many community service providers and the families, with more emphasis on opportunity and less upon punishment. In addition, the timing of early intervention may prove to be of considerable importance, and therefore we must modify our stance from reactive to proactive in order to attract the target population. Perhaps most important, an early intervention approach to child abuse must be flexible and responsive to the individual needs of the family. The teaching of skills and knowledge related to childrearing can best be accomplished when the unique attributes, values, and limitations of each family are fully understood (Cohn, 1982), and the goals are established in accordance with each family's relative needs.

REFERENCES

AINSWORTH, M. D. S. (1980). Attachment and child abuse. In G. Gerbner, C. J. Ross, & E. Zigler (Eds.), *Child abuse: An agenda for action*. New York: Oxford University Press.

AINSWORTH, M. D. S., BLEHAR, M., WATERS, E., & WALL, S. (1978). *Patterns of attachment: Observations in the strange situation at home*. Hillsdale, NJ: Erlbaum.

ALVY, K. T. (1975). Preventing child abuse. *American Psychologist, 30*, 921-928.

AMBROSE, S., HAZZARD, A., & HAWORTH, J. (1980). Cognitive-behavioral parenting groups for abusive families. *Child Abuse & Neglect, 4*, 119-125.

APPELBAUM, A. S. (1977). Developmental retardation in infants as a concomitant of physical child abuse. *Journal of Abnormal Child Psychology, 5*, 417-423.

ATWATER, J. B., & MORRIS, E. K. (1979). *Implications of child effects research for behavioral application*. Paper presented at the meeting of the American Psychological Association, New York.

BANDURA, A. (1973). *Aggression: A social learning analysis*. Englewood Cliffs, NJ: Prentice-Hall.

BELL, R. Q., & HARPER, L. (1977). *Child effects on adults*. Hillsdale, NJ: Erlbaum.

BELSKY, J. (1980). Child maltreatment: An ecological integration. *American Psychologist, 35*, 320-335.

BELSKY, J., GOODE, M. K., & MOST, R. K. (1980). Maternal stimulation and infant exploratory competence: Cross-sectional, correlational, and experimental analyses. *Child Development, 51*, 1163-1178.

BERKOWITZ, L. (1974). Some determinants of impulsive aggression: Role of mediated associations with reinforcement for aggression. *Psychological Review, 81*, 165-176.

BOLTON, F. G., LANER, R. H., & KANE, S. P. (1980). Child maltreatment risk among adolescent mothers. *American Journal of Orthopsychiatry, 50*, 489-504.

BRUNNQUELL, D., CRICHTON, L., & EGELAND, B. (1981). Maternal personality and attitude in disturbances of child rearing. *American Journal of Orthopsychiatry, 51*, 680-691.

BURGESS, R. L., & CONGER, R. (1978). Family interactions in abusive, neglectful, and normal families. *Child Development, 49*, 1163-1173.

BURGESS, R. L., & RICHARDSON, R. A. (1984). Coercive interpersonal contingencies as a determinant of child abuse: Implications for treatment and prevention. In R. F. Dangel & R. A. Polster (Eds.), *Behavioral parent training: Issues in research and practice*. New York: Guilford Press.

CAREW, J. (1979). Commentary: The Ypsilanti-Carnegie infant education project. *Monographs of the High/Scope Educational Research Foundation, 6*, 75-80.

COHN, A. H. (1982). Special report-stopping abuse before it occurs: Different solutions for different population groups. *Child Abuse and Neglect, 6*, 473-483.

DENICOLA, J., & SANDLER, J. (1980). Training abusive parents in cognitive-behavioral techniques. *Behavior Therapy, 11*, 263-270.

DIETRICH, K. N., STARR, R. H., & KAPLAN, M. G. (1980). Maternal stimulation and care of abused infants. In T. M. Field, S. Goldberg, R. Stern, & A. M. Sostek (Eds.),

High-risk infants and children: Adult and peer interactions. New York: Academic Press.

DOHRENWEND, B. S. (1978). Social stress and community psychology. *American Journal of Community Psychology, 6*, 1-14.

EGELAND, B., & SROUFE, L. A. (1981). Attachment and early maltreatment. *Child Development, 52*, 44-52.

EGELAND, B., & VAUGHN, B. (1981). Failure of "bond formation" as a cause of abuse, neglect, and maltreatment. *American Journal of Orthopsychiatry, 51*, 78-84.

ELMER, E. (1977). A follow-up study of traumatized children. *Pediatrics, 59*, 273-279.

EPSTEIN, A. S. (1980). *Assessing the child development information needed by adolescent parents with very young children.* (Project report). Ypsilanti, Michigan: High/Scope Educational Research Foundation.

FRIEDMAN, R., SANDLER, J., HERNANDEZ, M., & WOLFE, D. (1981). Child abuse. In E. Mash & L. Terdal (Eds.), *Behavioral assessment of childhood disorders.* New York: Guilford Press.

FRODI, A. M. (1981). Contribution of infant characteristics to child abuse. *American Journal of Mental Deficiency, 85*, 341-349.

FRODI, A. M., & LAMB, M. E. (1980). Child abusers' responses to infant smiles and cries. *Child Development, 51*, 238-241.

GAINES, R., SANDGRUND, A., GREEN, A. H., & POWER, E. (1978). Etiological factors in child maltreatment: A multivariate study of abusing, neglecting, and normal mothers. *Journal of Abnormal Psychology, 87*, 531-540.

GELLES, R. J., & STRAUS, M. A. (1979). Determinants of violence in the family: Toward a theoretical integration. In W. R. Burr, R. Hill, F. I. Nye, & I. L. Reiss (Eds.), *Contemporary theories about the family.* New York: Free Press.

HELFER, R. E. (1982). A review of the literature on the prevention of child abuse and neglect. *Child Abuse & Neglect, 6*, 251-261.

HOLAHAN, C. J., & SPEARLY, J. L. (1980). Coping and ecology: An integrative model for community psychology. *American Journal of Community Psychology, 8*, 671-685.

ISAACS, C. D. (1982). Treatment of child abuse: A review of the behavioral interventions. *Journal of Applied Behavior Analysis, 15*, 273-294.

KINARD, E. M., & KLERMAN, L. V. (1980). Teenage parenting and child abuse: Are they related? *American Journal of Orthopsychiatry, 50*, 481-488.

KNUTSON, J. F. (1978). Child abuse as an area of aggression research. *Journal of Pediatric Psychology, 3*, 20-27.

PARKE, R. D., & COLLMER, C. W. (1975). Child abuse: An interdisciplinary analysis. In E. M. Hetherington (Ed.), *Review of child development research* (Vol. 5). Chicago: University of Chicago Press.

PATTERSON, G. R. (1982). *Coercive family process.* Eugene, OR: Castalia.

PAWLBY, S. J., & HALL, F. (1980). Early interactions and later language development of children whose mothers come from disrupted families of origin. In T. M. Fields, S. Goldberg, R. Stern, & A. M. Sostek (Eds.), *High risk infants and children: Adult and peer interactions.* New York: Academic Press.

POLLOCK, C., & STEELE, B. (1972). A therapeutic approach to the parents. In C. H. Kempe & R. E. Helfer (Eds.), *Helping the battered child and his family.* Philadelphia: J. B. Lippincott.

REID, J. B., TAPLIN, P. S., & LORBER, R. (1981). A social interactional approach to the treatment of abusive families. In R. Stuart (Ed.), *Violent behavior: Social learning approaches to prediction, management, and treatment.* New York: Brunner/Mazel.

RULE, B. G., & NESDALE, A. R. (1976). Emotional arousal and aggressive behavior. *Psychological Bulletin, 83*, 851-863.

SPINETTA, J. J., & RIGLER, D. (1972). The child-abusing parent: A psychological review. *Psychological Bulletin, 77*, 296-304.

STANDING SENATE COMMITTEE ON HEALTH, WELFARE AND SCIENCE. (1980). *Child at risk.* Hull, Quebec: Minister of Supply and Services Canada.

STARR, R. H. (1982). A research-based approach to the prediction of child abuse. In R. H. Starr, Jr. (Ed.), *Child abuse prediction: Policy implications.* Cambridge, MA: Ballinger.

STEVENS-LONG, J. E. (1973). The effect of behavioral context on some aspects of adult disciplinary practice and effort. *Child Development, 44,* 476-484.

STRAIN, P. S., & SHORES, R. E. (1977). Social interaction development among behaviorally handicapped preschool children: Research and educational implications. *Psychology in the Schools, 14,* 300-311.

TORO, P. A. (1982). Developmental effects of child abuse: A review. *Child Abuse & Neglect, 6,* 423-431.

TULKIN, S. R., & COHLER, B. J. (1973). Childrearing attitudes and mother-child interaction in the first year of life. *Merrill-Palmer Quarterly, 19,* 95-106.

VASTA, R. (1982). Physical child abuse: A dual-component analysis. *Developmental Review, 2,* 125-149.

VASTA, R., & COPITCH, P. (1981). Simulating conditions of child abuse in the laboratory. *Child Development, 52,* 164-170.

WAHLER, R. G. (1980). The insular mother: Her problems in parent-child treatment. *Journal of Applied Behavior Analysis, 13,* 207-219.

WAHLER, R. G., & DUMAS, J. E. (in press). "A chip off the old block": Some interpersonal characteristics of coercive children across generations. In P. Strain (Ed.), *Children's social behavior: Development, assessment, and modification.* New York: Academic Press.

WHITE, R. (1959). Motivation reconsidered: The concept of competence. *Psychological Review, 66,* 297-331.

WOLFE, D.A. (in press). Child abusive parents: An empirical review. *Psychological Bulletin.*

WOLFE, D. A. (1983). *Early intervention methods for child abuse prevention.* Paper presented at the meeting of the American Psychological Association, Anaheim, CA.

WOLFE, D. A., FAIRBANK, J., KELLY, J. A., & BRADLYN, A. S. (1983). Child abusive parents' physiological responses to stressful and non-stressful behavior in children. *Behavioral Assessment, 5,* 363-371.

WOLFE, D. A. & MOSK, M. D. (1983). Behavioral comparisons of children from abusive and distressed families. *Journal of Consulting and Clinical Psychology, 51,* 702-708.

WOLFE, D. A., & SANDLER, J. (1981). Training abusive parents in effective child management. *Behavior Modification, 5,* 320-335.

WOLFE, D. A., SANDLER, J., & KAUFMAN, K. (1981). A competency-based parent training program for child abusers. *Journal of Consulting and Clinical Psychology, 49,* 633-640.

WOLFE, D. A., ST. LAWRENCE, J., GRAVES, K., BREHONY, K., BRADLYN, D., & KELLY, J. A. (1982). Intensive behavioral parent training for a child abusive mother. *Behavior Therapy, 13,* 438-451.

10

The Social Behavior of Hyperactive Children: Developmental Changes, Drug Effects, and Situational Variation

RUSSELL A. BARKLEY

Hyperactive children, or those having Attention Deficit Disorder with Hyperactivity (American Psychiatric Association, 1980), are characterized by their inattentiveness, proneness to distractability, impulsiveness, restlessness or overactivity, and difficulties with restricting their behavior as a situation demands (Barkley, 1981, 1982; Ross & Ross, 1982; Routh, 1980). Problems with sustained attention, particularly to activities lacking intrinsic appeal, and impulsive responding, are believed to be the sine qua non of the disorder (Douglas, 1980; Douglas & Peters, 1979). These symptoms appear to arise quite early in childhood, often by two to three years of age, and seem to be relatively pervasive in their effects on the child's adaptive functioning

The research projects detailed herein were supported in part by grant number MH 32334-01 from the National Institutes of Health to the author and by funds provided by the Department of Neurology, Medical College of Wisconsin.

across a variety of situations (Barkley, 1982). Follow-up studies suggest that while symptoms of motor overactivity and restlessness may decline with age, as they do in normal children (Routh, Schroeder, & O'Tuama, 1974), difficulties with inattention, lack of concentration, impulsivity, and peer relationship problems persist in these children well into their young adult years (see Ross & Ross, 1982; Weiss, Hechtman, & Perlman, 1978).

While environmental theories of hyperactivity are not taken seriously by most investigators, a role for environmental factors should not be completely discounted. Substantial evidence suggests that they may play some part in modulating the expression and severity of the disorder, as well as the development of secondary symptoms, such as depression and low self-esteem. No one questions the fact that the child's behavior and symptoms are displayed relative to some social context and some significant individuals (parents, teachers, peers), but there appears to have been a lack of interest in these social contexts and their effects on behavior until the mid to late 1970s. Yet, the very fact that the child is referred by adults for clinical services indicates that the child's behavior by itself is not the problem, but that it is the child's conflict with his social environment that results in his being identified as deviant from normal children. Clearly greater study of these social contexts is warranted.

The present chapter will review several investigations conducted in our clinic and laboratory at the Medical College of Wisconsin that focused on the interface between the child, his symptoms and characteristics, and the social context in which he interacts, especially his interactions with his parents.

The first report of parent-child interactions of overactive children appears to have been conducted by Battle and Lacey (1972), utilizing parent reports collected during the Fels Longitudinal Studies. The children were not clinically identified as hyperactive, partly because the diagnosis was not especially widespread at that time. They were selected instead on the basis of parents' descriptions of excessive activity in the children. The mothers of the overactive boys were found to be more disapproving, unaffectionate, critical, and severe in their punishment of the boys than the mothers of non-hyperactive children. The overactive boys were themselves described as less compliant, more attention-seeking, and requiring greater supervision than their normally active peers.

Within the next several years, Campbell reported two studies which directly observed and recorded the interactions of clinically diagnosed hyperactive children with their mothers in a laboratory setting. In her 1973 study, Campbell compared the mother-child interactions among hyperactive, impulsive, and reflective children during a task accomplishment situation. The difficulty of the tasks was varied, and the results indicated that on the relatively easy tasks, there were few, if any, differences among the groups. However, the mothers of hyperactive children gave their children considerably more help and encouragement during the more difficult tasks than did the mothers of the two other groups. Although the results could not permit the drawing of direct causal statements from these data, Campbell speculated that the additional supervision and control provided by the mothers of hyperactive children probably were reactions to the child's difficulties with concentration, impulsiveness, and distractibility. In a somewhat similar study, Campbell (1975) compared the interactions of hyperactive, learning disabled, and normal boys with their mothers. The results generally replicated the earlier findings in showing hyperactive children to be less compliant, in need of more direct help and encouragement, and to be more attention-seeking than the other groups of boys. These studies provide the first direct glimpse of the interaction conflicts of hyperactive children with others.

Our initial study of hyperactive and normal children with their mothers (Cunningham & Barkley, 1979) utilized hyperactive boys who had been identified as such by their pediatricians and who were receiving stimulant medication for control of their symptoms. The boys were observed individually with their mothers during both a free play and task accomplishment period. The Response-Class Matrix (Mash, Terdal, & Anderson, 1973) was used to record the interaction sequences. This system requires two highly trained observers who simultaneously code the mother's responses to the child's behavior and the child's responses to her behaviors. That is, one coder scores the mother's behavior as an antecedent using seven different behavior categories, and then records the child's reactions to her behavior in at least six different behavior categories. The other coder scores the opposite relationship, that being the child's behavior as the antecedent and the mother's reaction to those child behaviors (see Barkley, 1981). This system permits, to some extent, the computation of contingent, reciprocal relations within the interaction patterns.

The results indicated, similar to those of Campbell, that hyperactive boys were significantly less compliant to their mothers' requests, and were more negative than normal boys in both the free play and task settings. The mothers of the hyperactive boys gave significantly more commands and were more negative to the boys than to normal children. Although these interaction differences could be detected during the free play situation, they became more salient, frequent, and negative during the task period when mothers were required to accomplish at least five different tasks with their hyperactive boys. Interestingly, during free play, when the hyperactive boys initiated interactions with their mothers, the mothers were less likely to respond to these social initiatives than were the mothers of normal boys. A similar pattern of diminished responsiveness to social initiatives was also seen in the reactions of hyperactive boys to their mothers' interactions. While our initial clinical impressions were that the mothers reacted this way to the hyperactive children simply in an effort to control their exuberant and obstreperous behavior, the data would not permit such a formal conclusion on the direction of effects in the interactions.

We therefore conducted a double-blind, drug-placebo study on these hyperactive boys utilizing Ritalin (methylphenidate) in doses comparable to those prescribed for the children prior to this study (Barkley & Cunningham, 1979). A cross-over design was used, with each child serving as his own control. Children remained in each of the drug conditions (drug or placebo) for one week, were observed at the end of that week in the clinic playroom, and then crossed over to the opposite drug condition after which the second observation occurred. Our results indicated that Ritalin significantly increased the compliance of the hyperactive children with their mothers' commands during both free play and task situations, resulting in a decline in the number of commands given by the mothers. The mothers also behaved less negatively towards their children and responded more to their interactions when the children were on medication as opposed to placebo. The results clearly suggested that the high level of commands and negative interactions of the mothers towards their hyperactive children was, to a great extent, a reaction to the inattentive, off-task, and noncompliant behavior of the hyperactive children, rather than being a major cause of it. This did not rule out the possibility that the mothers' directive and negative interactions could not eventually come to exacerbate the behavioral difficulties of the hyperactive child.

These initial results raised a variety of questions, chief among them being the extent to which these interaction patterns might change with age and how differing doses of medication might affect these developmental patterns.

SUBJECTS AND PROCEDURES

All hyperactive children used in our studies were boys, ages three to 12 years, of at least average intelligence, and without evidence of brain damage, epilepsy, autism, psychosis, aphasia, or sensory deficits. They were diagnosed hyperactive based upon parent complaints of inattention, restlessness, and poor impulse control with onset prior to age six years and a duration of problems for at least 12 months. Additionally, the children had to score two standard deviations above the mean on both the Conners Parent Symptom Questionnaire (see Goyette, Conners, & Ulrich, 1978) and the Werry-Weiss-Peters Activity Rating Scale (see Barkley, 1981). The children also had to be rated by parents as problematic in eight of 16 situations in the home using the Home Situations Questionnaire (Barkley, 1981).

The children were observed in a clinic playroom during a free play and task period while interacting with their mothers. Interactions were recorded using the Response Class Matrix (Mash et al., 1973). Children were removed from stimulant medications at least 24 hours prior to the observations or for the entire length of the drug-placebo conditions in the case of the drug studies described below.

DEVELOPMENTAL EFFECTS ON PARENT-CHILD INTERACTIONS

One of the first variables of interest was whether the age of the child was related to any differences in the interactions of hyperactive and normal children. The initial study of developmental changes in the parent-child interactions of hyperactive children (Barkley, Karlsson, Strzelecki, & Murphy, 1984) employed 54 hyperactive children ranging from four years-one month to nine years-11 months of age. These 54 hyperactive children were divided into three groups of 18 subjects on the basis of age. The youngest group consisted of children between the ages of four years-one month and five years-11 months, while the older hyperactive group consisted of children from eight years-zero months of age to nine years-11 months. The middle group was six years-zero months to seven years-11 months of age. The three groups were not significantly different with respect to intelligence, maternal age, or scores on the Conners Questionnaire, the Werry-Weiss-Peters Activity Rating Scale, or the Home Situations Questionnaire. All mothers were the biological parents of the hyperactive children or had adopted the children shortly after birth. None of the mothers were foster parents or recent adoptive parents.

In the free play situation the youngest hyperactive children initiated more social interactions with their mothers than the older hyperactive children. The mothers of the youngest children asked more questions of their children as compared to the mothers of older hyperactive children. The pattern suggests that with age, older hyperactive children play more independently of their mothers while initiating fewer interactions toward their mothers. In turn, with increasing age of the child, the mothers decrease the number of questions they ask.

The task situation revealed more difficulties in the children's behavior than was seen in free play, and the differences between the youngest and older hyperactive children became more salient. Mothers of the youngest hyperactive children gave nearly twice as many commands to their children than was seen in the older hyperactive groups. The youngest hyperactive children were also significantly less compliant with those commands and likely to sustain their compliance for a significantly shorter duration. Finally, even when the hyperactive children complied with commands, mothers of the youngest hyperactives were more likely to respond to this compliance with further commands and negative behavior as compared to the reactions of mothers of older hyperactive children. Thus, the interaction conflicts of hyperactive children with their mothers appear to improve to some extent with increasing age of the children.

Next, a large-scale study was undertaken comparing the mother-child interactions of hyperactive and normal children across five different age levels (year levels five-nine). There were 60 hyperactive children and 60 normal children, with 12 children in each group at each of the five year levels. The results of this large-scale investigation are reported in greater detail elsewhere (Barkley, Karlsson, & Pollard, in press). The interaction data were submitted to two-way analyses of covariance (group by age level) with the child's intellectual estimate, the mother's age, and the mother's educational level serving as the covariates. The means and standard deviations for the hyperactive and normal children on each interaction measure collapsed across age levels are displayed in Table 1 along with the results from the statistical analyses.

As we found in our earlier studies, the free play period was not as evocative of behavior problems in children as the task period. Nonetheless, some group differences in free play emerged and generally

TABLE 1
Measures of Mother-Child Interactions During Free Play and Task for
Both Hyperactive and Normal Children

Measure	Hyperactive Mean	S.D.	Normal Mean	S.D.	Group* $p <$	Age* $p <$
FREE PLAY PERIOD:						
Mother Initiates Interaction	56.6	13.6	65.3	16.8	.01	—
Child Responds	85.9	8.7	87.8	10.8	—	—
Mother Questions	9.7	5.2	10.1	7.4	—	—
Child Responds	84.9	16.2	89.8	17.4	—	—
Mother's No Response Percent	25.7	14.3	21.0	17.6	—	—
Mother's Reward Percent	1.6	3.5	1.2	2.6	—	—
Mother's Command Percent	6.6	5.9	3.2	3.3	—	.10
Child Complies	81.6	27.6	90.1	21.7	.01	.05
Mother's Negative Behavior	0.7	2.0	1.7	12.9	.05	—
Child Initiates Interaction	71.2	15.3	79.5	19.5	.01	—
Mother Responds	82.8	8.2	88.7	6.9	.01	—
Child's No Response Percent	0.4	0.9	2.2	12.5	.01	—
Child's Negative Behavior	0.6	1.5	0.1	0.7	.01	—
Child's Independent Play	26.4	15.2	17.6	16.1	.01	—
Mother Attends to Play	32.0	19.0	36.0	28.0	—	—
Mother Controls Play	7.3	10.5	2.4	7.8	.01	.10

TASK.PERIOD:						
Mother Initiates Interaction	42.2	15.9	58.1	13.7	.01	.05
Mother Questions	6.4	7.3	7.0	5.7	—	—
Mother's No Response Percent	15.5	10.4	12.8	9.2	.10	.01
Mother's Reward Percent	2.6	3.0	2.8	3.0	—	—
Mother's Command Percent	32.1	16.1	19.8	10.7	.01	.01
Child Complies	90.0	12.1	96.8	5.9	.01	.05
Mother's Negative Behavior	2.4	2.8	0.5	0.9	.01	—
Mean Compliance Duration**	4.4	2.9	6.9	3.7	.01	.01
Child's Compliance Percent	89.1	9.1	97.8	3.3	.01	.01
Mother Responds Positively to Compliance	52.9	16.0	69.6	11.9	.01	.05
Mother Responds Negatively to Compliance	32.8	15.9	19.1	10.1	.01	.01
Child's Competing Behavior (Noncompliance)	8.6	7.6	1.7	2.8	.01	—
Mother Responds Positively to Competing	27.7	30.6	31.6	43.5	—	—
Mother Responds Negatively to Competing	49.9	37.1	23.6	39.0	.01	.10
Child's Negative Behavior	1.9	3.1	0.6	1.4	.01	—

*Refers to the statistical significance level of the main effect for this factor (Group or Age) in the analysis of covariance.
**All measures reported in the table are percentages or conditional percentages of occurrence except this one. Mean Compliance Duration refers to the number of intervals in which the child's behavior was scored as compliance divided by the number of intervals during which the mother gave a command. Hence it is actually the average number of intervals of child compliance per maternal command.

parallel the results found in our initial studies. The results in Table 1 for free play suggest that hyperactive children were significantly less compliant with their mothers' commands than were normal children. The hyperactive children also initiated fewer general interactions with their mothers, demonstrated somewhat greater negative behavior during free play, and preferred to play independently of their mothers more than was seen in the normal mother-child dyads. As in our previous studies, the mothers of hyperactive boys initiated fewer interactions toward the children, and were less responsive to their children's interactions when the children chose to initiate them. Instead, mothers of hyperactive children spent more time giving commands to the children. In fact, they gave twice as many commands as the mothers of normal children, despite the fact that this was to have been a free play, non-directive situation. As noted above, the hyperactive children spent more time involved in playing independently of their mothers. But when play occurred, the mothers of hyperactive children were nearly three times as likely to respond with control of the play through the use of commands, negative statements, or direction as compared to the mothers of normal children. Clearly, the mothers of hyperactive children find their children's play and interactions during free play to be less appropriate than is seen in normal parent-child interactions. There were no significant effects for age on the free play interaction measures.

During the task period, more differences between the groups emerged, and the differences themselves were more salient. As in free play, the mothers of hyperactive children initiated significantly fewer interactions toward their children but spent almost twice as much time giving commands to the children as compared to mothers of normal children. The mothers were also more likely to engage in negative behavior toward the child during the task accomplishment. The children were found to be significantly less compliant with maternal commands and to remain on-task for a significantly shorter duration of compliance than were the normal children. As expected, the hyperactive children were more likely to engage in behavior which competed with maternal requests, underscoring the oppositional nature of this group. Yet, even when the children did comply, the mothers of hyperactive children were less likely to respond positively to the child's compliance and were more likely to respond with commands, negative behavior, and control than was seen in the normal mother-child dyads. This intimates that these mothers found the child's compliance to be of a significantly inferior quality than that seen in normal children, necessitating greater control and supervision in order to see that the tasks were accomplished. Likewise, when the hyperactive children were engaged in competing or off-task behavior, their mothers were twice as likely to respond with control and direction than were the mothers of normal children.

There were also a number of main effects for age on the interaction measures during the task period. These are displayed in Table 2.

The results indicate that mothers initiate more interactions toward their six- and eight-year-old children than to their five- and nine-year-olds. Mothers also seem to spend a greater amount of time in "no response" or simply passively observing the behavior of their children as the children increase in age. There is a corresponding decline in the number of commands given to children as age increases, which parallels an increase in the amount of compliance of the children with age. The children were also found to improve in their ability to sustain compliance to requests with increasing age. Perhaps related to the improvements in child compliance, the mothers were less likely to respond negatively to the compliance of their children with increasing age levels of the child. All of these results suggest that as children age, they become more compliant and better able to sustain compliance to requests. In response, mothers decrease their commands to these children while spending more time engaged in general social interactions or simply passive observance of the child. In short, as children develop greater self-control and management over their own behavior, mothers decrease their control of the children. Because of the lack of group by age interactions, these conclusions apply to both hyperactive and normal children.

EFFECTS OF STIMULANT MEDICATION

My earlier studies suggested that Ritalin, and perhaps the stimulant drugs in general, produce significant effects on the social interactions of hyperactive children toward their mothers, and that mothers show a collateral change in their behavior as their children's behavior improves. I was sufficiently intrigued by this finding to wonder whether these drug effects were dose related, and whether the effects of the medications varied with age of the child. And so, as part of the large-scale developmental study described above, the 60 hyperactive children who participated in that study subsequently were involved in a double-blind, drug-placebo experiment examining the effects of two doses of Ritalin (0.3 mg/kg/dose b.i.d. and 0.7 mg/kg/dose b.i.d.). The procedures

TABLE 2

Measures of Mother-Child Interactions for Hyperactive and Normal Boys
Across Five Age Levels of Boys

Interaction Measures From Task Period	Means for Each Age Level				
	5	6	7	8	9
Mother Initiates Interaction					
Overall	43.9	54.2	50.0	56.6	46.0
Hyperactives	33.8	49.3	38.9	47.4	41.5
Normals	54.1	59.0	61.0	65.8	50.4
Mother's No Response Percent					
Overall	7.7	11.7	15.4	12.2	23.7
Hyperactives	9.4	11.6	19.8	12.3	24.4
Normals	6.0	11.8	10.9	12.1	23.0
Mother's Command Percent					
Overall	39.1	24.3	24.9	21.6	19.9
Hyperactives	47.3	29.1	31.0	30.1	23.0
Normals	30.8	19.4	18.8	13.1	16.8
Child's Compliance					
Overall	89.2	91.3	96.6	94.6	95.1
Hyperactives	84.3	88.1	94.8	90.1	92.2
Normals	94.1	94.5	98.3	99.1	97.9

Mean Compliance Duration					
Overall	3.6	5.2	4.8	7.7	6.8
Hyperactives	2.5	4.6	3.5	5.8	5.5
Normals	4.7	5.7	6.1	9.5	8.1
Mother Responds Positively to Child's Compliance					
Overall	56.9	63.9	57.9	68.1	59.3
Hyperactives	45.8	58.8	46.1	59.7	53.9
Normals	68.0	68.9	69.6	76.5	64.7
Mother Responds Negatively to Child's Compliance					
Overall	37.7	24.5	26.7	21.2	20.0
Hyperactives	48.0	28.8	34.0	29.1	24.2
Normals	27.3	20.2	19.3	13.3	15.8

used to observe and record the parent-child interactions remained identical to those discussed above. The experimental design was therefore a five (age levels) by three (placebo, low dose, high dose) factorial design with repeated measures on the second factor (drug level). The children were randomly assigned within age level to one of the six possible drug orders.

The results of this study are reported in greater detail elsewhere (Barkley, Karlsson, Pollard, & Murphy, in press). In general, there were virtually no effects of the medication on free play interactions. As with our previous research, drug effects were much more apparent during the task situation. Most of the drug effects were related to the high dose of Ritalin as compared to the placebo condition. The high dose of Ritalin (0.7 mg/kg/dose given twice daily) resulted in increased interactions initiated by the mothers toward their hyperactive children as well as decreased commands given to the children. Ritalin also resulted in improvements in child compliance, and here the two doses differed somewhat, with the low dose producing no difference from placebo, and the high dose being significantly more effective than either the placebo or low dose of medication. Improvements were also seen in the duration of the children's compliance per command (sustained compliance) with both doses of medication producing significant effects but a greater effect produced by the high dose condition. In response to these improvements in child behavior, the mothers of hyperactive children decreased their control and negative reactions toward the children's compliance. This suggests that the quality of the child's compliance and behavior may also have improved with the administration of Ritalin, especially the high dose of medication. Both doses of medication significantly improved the child's behavior in the home as measured by the Home Situations Questionnaire (Barkley, 1981), but again there was no difference between the two doses in their effectiveness in this regard.

Both doses of medication produced increases in the number of side effects experienced by the children, but the doses were not significantly different in this regard. There also appeared to be no increase in the severity of those side effects that were noted by the use of the higher dose of Ritalin.

This large-scale drug study appears to demonstrate, as our earlier research had, that Ritalin is likely to produce greater changes in hyperactive behavior and parent-child interactions during the task situations as opposed to free play. The improvements appear to be those involved in better child compliance and better sustained compliance to commands. As a result, the mothers of hyperactive children provide fewer commands to the children, initiate more positive and general interactions toward the children, and decrease their negative responding to the children's lack of compliance and off-task behavior. There was little evidence for a differential effect of the two doses, although the high dose produced a greater number of significant improvements than the low dose in the interaction measures. Nonetheless, on the basis of parent ratings of home behavior, both doses appear to be equally effective in reducing problem behaviors in that environment.

There were virtually no main effects for age nor were there any interactions of age with drug effects during the free play situation. But, again, there were several main effects for age regardless of drug condition witnessed during the task situation. These findings were virtually identical to those seen in the earlier study. There were also no significant age by treatment interactions suggesting that the effects of medication were similar across all age groups of the children.

SITUATIONAL VARIATION IN HYPERACTIVE BEHAVIOR

Hyperactive children were generally better behaved in the clinic playroom situation than they were in their home environments, as revealed in parent ratings of child behavior. In addition, within the clinic playroom situation, hyperactive children were more discernible from normal children during the task situation as opposed to free play. The changes observed in the parent-child interactions with the increasing age of the children were also more likely to be revealed within task situations than free play settings, and the same conclusions could be said for the effects of medication on the child's behavior. Obviously, hyperactive children do not misbehave at the same level or the same rate in every situation, but seem to have their greatest difficulties in situations requiring restriction of their behavior, compliance with commands or rules, and sustained effort toward a task. It was therefore of interest to determine whether similar fluctuations occurred in the social behavior of hyperactive children across differing situations within the home.

I randomly selected, from the records of all the hyperactive children involved in our studies to date, the reports of parents for 30 of the hyperactive children and 30 matched controls. The responses to the Home Situations Questionnaire were then tabulated and analyzed. From this analysis I could determine, within the limits of parental report data, the percentage of hyperactive children posing problems in the situations described on the Home Situations Questionnaire as well as the severity rating given to these problems. Some of the results are set forth in Table 3, which displays the percentage of hyperactive children having problems in each of 14 situations listed on the Home Situations Questionnaire as compared to the percentage of normal children having problems in those settings.

Parents were permitted to rate the severity of the behavior problem within each situation using a scale from 1 (mild) to 9 (severe); the mean severity scores are also displayed in Table 3. Analyses of variance comparing these severity scores indicated that in every one of these 14 situations, hyperactive children were rated as presenting significantly more severe problems compared to their normal peers. Table 3 suggests that, although hyperactive children present more problems in all situations compared to normal children, the frequency of children having problems and the mean severity fluctuates to some extent with the nature of the situation. The greatest difficulties for hyperactive children appear in situations involving other people, such as when the child must play with others, when visitors are in the home, when visiting other people, or when the parent is in a public place such as stores or restaurants. Problems also occur more often in situations requiring some degree of restraint on the part of the child, such as during parent conversations on the telephone and mealtimes. While at least 75% of the hyperactive children presented problems when their fathers were at home, these problems were the least severe among the 14 situations shown in Table 3. This seems to underscore parent reports that the children are somewhat better behaved for their fathers than their mothers.

These results suggested what had already been demonstrated in the clinic playroom situations. When hyperactive children are required to restrict their behavior in accordance with situational demands, commands of others, or rules of social conduct, they have greater difficulties with their behavior compared to normal children, and compared to situations where there are few restraints on their behavior, e.g., playing alone or during bath times.

DISCUSSIONS AND CONCLUSIONS

The results of the studies reviewed above permit a number of conclusions and implications to be drawn about Attention Deficit Disorder

TABLE 3

Percentage of Hyperactive and Normal Children Displaying Problems in 14 Home Situations and the Mean Severity Rating in Each Setting

Situation	Hyperactive		Normal	
	Percent	Mean Severity*	Percent	Mean Severity*
While Playing Alone	40.0	4.3	0.0	0.0
Playing with Others	90.0	5.4	10.0	1.6
Mealtimes	86.7	4.7	13.3	3.0
Getting Dressed	73.3	6.1	10.0	2.3
Washing/Bathing	43.3	5.1	16.7	1.2
When Parent is on Phone	93.3	6.6	33.3	1.3
While Watching Television	80.0	5.0	3.3	2.0
When Visitors are in Home	96.7	6.1	30.0	1.6
When Visiting Others	96.7	5.4	13.3	1.5
Public Places	96.7	5.4	23.3	2.7
When Father is at Home	73.3	3.9	6.7	2.5
When Asked to do Chores	86.7	5.6	36.7	2.0
At Bedtime	83.3	5.0	20.0	1.5
While Riding in the Car	73.3	4.8	20.0	1.7

*Severity was rated by parents on a scale from 1 (mild) to 9 (severe)

with Hyperactivity in children, and these will be discussed below under separate sections dealing with theoretical, methodological, and clinical implications. As is customary, all of these implications must be viewed in the context that they are simply initial findings which require further study and replication before greater confidence can be placed in them.

Theoretical Implications

While the biological correlates and causes of hyperactivity are becoming increasingly accepted by serious investigators in this field, this hardly rules out the effects of environmental factors which may influence the expression and modulation of the child's symptoms, their severity, and the development of secondary or related symptoms over time. Such environmental factors may also determine the nature of the interaction conflicts which the child experiences with other social agents, particularly parents and teachers. We cannot forget that, to some degree, the unique characteristics of the parent or teacher dictate the way in which child behaviors will be responded to by the individual. The studies described above suggest that the primary symptoms of the hyperactive child, such as inattentiveness, poor concentration, and impulsivity, clearly lead the child into conflict with others in his social environment, resulting in his behavior being judged as inappropriate with environmental expectations and demands. The environment then reacts with various control strategies in an effort to constrain to some extent the child's quantitatively or qualitatively inappropriate behaviors. While such control strategies may not be completely successful, they do influence the subsequent responses of the child to his environment.

More specifically, if one examines the differences in the behavior of hyperactive children in these studies under varying social circumstances, one cannot help but be impressed with the fact that those settings that require greater demands of the child for restraint, self-control, and sustained goal-directed behavior are the settings in which hyperactive children will be much more distinguishable from their normal peers. Such situations seem to tax the very essence of the deficiency (or deficiencies) in the hyperactive child, thereby shedding greater light on the nature of the disorder. From the clinic playroom interaction data, it appears that free play situations, especially those involving the sole attention of the parent to the child in a small playroom setting, do not pose great difficulty for the hyperactive child compared to normal children. It was repeatedly demonstrated that in these situations, the hyperactive child is not especially distinguishable from his normal peers, with the exception of being slightly less compliant with parent requests, and spending somewhat greater time involved in play independent of the mother as opposed to involving her. While these differences from normal were statistically significant, the difference between the absolute levels of occurrence on these measures are not especially striking, indicating substantial overlap of the behavioral distributions of hyperactive with normal children. This suggests that on a case-by-case basis, in free play settings, observers might have great difficulty reliably separating the hyperactive from the normal child.

In contrast, the settings involving the accomplishment of tasks by the child under the direction of the parent lead to more salient and obvious distinctions between the hyperactive and normal samples. In this situation, the hyperactive children were more noncompliant, spent more time competing with requests (off-task behavior), and were unable to sustain their compliance with requests for as long a time as normal children. Apparently in response to these difficulties, the parents of these hyperactive children responded with greater commands to the child, greater direction and supervision of his compliance, and more negative behavior as shown in greater warnings, threats, yelling, and sometimes disciplining of the child.

Earlier research suggested that these may be the difficulties which bring hyperactive children to child guidance centers for assistance and which prove the most irritating and frustrating to their parents (see Barkley & Cunningham, 1980). These earlier studies, and those by Routh and Schroeder (1976), found that the standard child behavior rating scales employed with hyperactive children correlate significantly and substantially with playroom measures of noncompliance as opposed to measures of activity level or attention span. In other words, it is not simply the child's inattentiveness, impulsiveness and restlessness alone that result in the referral, but the effects that they have on the child's social interactions with others that proves so distressing to their care-givers, thereby leading to referral for treatment. Research continues to support the notion that alongside the well-recognized triad of primary problems of the hyperactive child (inattention, impulsivity, and restlessness) might also be placed the other primary social deficits of noncompliance, poor self-control, and an inability to sustain performance towards a goal comparable to same-age children.

These problems with compliance, self-control, and goal-directed be-

havior might all be subsumed under the concept of rule-governed behavior (Skinner, 1953). By this term is meant the ability of language
and rules to control behavior as opposed to that control exerted by
stimuli in the immediately surrounding environment. I have elsewhere
developed this idea more fully (Barkley, 1981), but it should be noted
here that there is a growing body of literature on the control of child
behavior by language in general, and the complex language and problem-solving deficiencies in hyperactive children in particular (see
Douglas, 1980) that supports its inclusion. In short, not only do hyperactive children have a deficit in their ability to "stop, look and
listen" as Douglas (1972) has so eloquently argued, but they are also
deficient in their ability to "do as we say, not as we do."

Our research also provides some implications for the understanding
of parent-child interactions in general. These studies suggest that parent and child behaviors seem closely locked to each other in a feedback
loop arrangement such that changes in child behavior produce almost
immediate changes in parental responses. While this supports much
of what Bell (1968, 1981), his colleagues (Bell & Harper, 1977), and
others (Lytton, 1979) have described in great detail elsewhere, some
of these findings do not. Bell indicated that while parent responses in
these interactions are in part a reaction to the child's immediate behavior, they may also be partly related to expectations, rules, and
standards to which the parent ascribes. The parent may have certain
notions about the manner in which he or she should respond to a child's
behavior and these expectations might govern the parent's responses
to a greater extent than simply the child's immediate behavior. The
present results do not seem to support this idea in that when child
behavior changed, either as a function of medication, setting demands,
or age, parent reactions also changed. In those studies where the
change in child behavior was produced immediately by medication or
a switch in situational demands, parent behaviors also changed immediately in virtual tandem with the child's behavioral changes. This
does not completely rule out the notion of a "thinking parent" as described by Bell, but suggests that parent behaviors are not quite so
slow to change in response to changes in child behavior as the "thinking
parent" concept might have one believe. It is possible that later changes
in parent behavior toward the child might well occur beyond the time
periods studied in our research as parents begin to shift their expectations and stereotypes of the child to be more consistent with the
newly developed, appropriate child behaviors.

In a different vein, these changes in child behavior and related changes in maternal response indicate that as the child's compliance and self-control improve, less control is exerted by the social environment. The environment recedes in its control to the extent that the child's development permits. As was demonstrated in the developmental studies of hyperactive and normal children, the behavior of both groups of children appears to improve with age, especially their compliance, and there is a corresponding decrease in the number of commands and amount of control displayed by the mother toward the child's behavior. The social environment seems to envelop the child's behavior in control, direction, and supervision on a level keeping with the child's current developmental abilities to restrain and control his own behavior. As the child's capacity for self-control and sustained performance toward a goal improves, control by the social environment is retracted to a similar degree. Such an interplay of a child's capacities with the social environment's responses is nothing short of fascinating.

Unfortunately, the research described above also suggests that for hyperactive children, there exists a chronic lag in the development of compliance and self-control relative to same-age normal peers, necessitating control over the child for longer periods of time than with normal children. It may prove to be this requirement for prolonged and greater supervision and control over the child that leads to strain in the parent-child relationship, perhaps stressing in some cases an already overtaxed parent. The developmental studies suggest, at least within the age limits explored here, that the hyperactive child shows a developmental pattern similar to that of normal children but one which never catches up to normal children. More recent follow-up studies of hyperactive children (see Weiss et al., 1978) indicate that even in young adulthood, hyperactive individuals remain distinguishable from their normal peers in their ability to sustain attention, inhibit responding, and demonstrate self-control. It seems doubtful that these hyperactive children ever catch up with normal children.

Some theorists (Willis & Lovaas, 1977), and certainly clinical lore, imply that the directive, negative, and controlling behaviors of the parents toward their hyperactive child may well have led to the development of the child's hyperactivity and poor self-control. The results from the drug studies described above do not support this view. If the fault or the deficiency in the interaction rests with the parents then altering the child's behavior should not result in any substantial changes in the parents' reactions to the child. However, if the parents' behavior toward the child is primarily a reaction to the child's characteristics and deficiencies in his behavior, then improving the child's characteristics or deficiencies should result in substantial change in maternal behavior. The findings from the drug studies, as well as the differences in hyperactive behavior between free play and task settings, support the latter interpretation. All of this suggests that, in large part, parental behaviors towards the hyperactive child are reactions to the child's inability to comply with situational demands, and not necessarily the cause of the child's lack of self-control.

This does not mean, however, that the mother's excessive supervision and control of the child might not lead to further difficulties in the child's behavior in the long run. Our research suggests that parents do not remain static in their efforts to control deviant behavior, but evolve through a hierarchy of possible control strategies which, if unsuccessful, might lead to actual physical disciplining of the child, and failing this, even incomplete acquiescence to the child's inappropriate behavior. Our observations parallel the findings of Patterson (1976) that parent and child negative behaviors escalate, perhaps in an effort to gain some control over the coercive responses of the other. These parental control reactions are apparently natural and even successful responses to the occasional excessive behavior of the normal child, but if displayed chronically may lead to exacerbation of the child's behavioral difficulties, and a deterioration in the overall parent-child relationship.

Methodological Implications

The series of studies described herein experienced several methodological problems that are well worth reviewing, if only to prevent others from repeating the same mistakes. One such difficulty occurred with the coding system itself. While differences between groups were detected using the Response Class Matrix, and drug effects were certainly noted during the stimulant drug research, it was our impression that the coding system lacked the specificity necessary for detecting precisely those behaviors which parents found irritating and necessary to control. The child's inappropriate behavior could be coded into only competing behavior (noncompliance or off-task behavior) or in the negative category (yelling, screaming, tantrums, etc.). Other types of behavior were obviously irritating to the parents and inappropriate, yet they might be classified in the categories of compliance or general interactions, and hence not be viewed as disruptive in the final computation of each dependent measure. This is not to say that the concept of the Response Class Matrix is not an effective way of coding behavior.

The problem seems to be that the behavior categories themselves could be more specific and perhaps more categories used in an effort to capture the essence of the hyperactive behavior. It was clear from the above studies that the coding system was capturing quantitative changes in child behavior, but in many cases did not capture qualitative aspects of the behavior, and these may be important aspects that the parents are responding to in their reactions to their children.

It was also clear from our research that the playroom environment was not as provocative of behavior problems in the hyperactive children as had been the playroom used in the initial studies. Since the procedures themselves were the same with respect to instructions to parents and the tasks to be done by the children, it can only be the physical parameters of the room which inhibited the children's hyperactive behavior and noncompliance. The playroom used in the present series of studies was approximately one-third the size of that used in the earlier studies. It may prove to be that the size of the playroom is a significant parameter in helping to elicit inappropriate behavior from hyperactive children.

Another difficulty with our procedure is that each child was observed in a one-to-one situation with his mother in a novel clinic playroom. Parents and teachers often indicate that hyperactive children are significantly better behaved when they are in a situation where they have the undivided attention of a single adult. One way to elicit further behavior problems would be to introduce a second adult to the playroom, or even a second child, which would force the hyperactive child to share the attention of the parent with someone else. As the results from the Home Situations Questionnaire revealed in several of our studies, one of the most problematic situations for hyperactive children is when they must share the attention of their parents with others, as is seen in situations where company is visiting the family, when a parent must talk on the telephone, or when other children are involved.

During some of our studies, parents suggested that in order to elicit greater deviant behavior in their children, the playroom might be equipped with more attractive toys, games, or activities that would likely be found within the typical individual's home. Such distractors as television, electronic games or video games, or highly attractive toys might be sufficient to distract the hyperactive child away from tasks more so than would be seen in normal children. The idea seems to be a good one, and would be worth exploring in future research of this sort.

It is possible that these problems give us some clue as to the types of difficulties the hyperactive child might be having. Parents would joke with our research assistants that we had found a cure for hyperactivity simply by placing the children within our small playroom. Given that the hyperactive child's behavior in his natural environment was so deviant, one might question precisely what it was about our playroom or our procedures that achieved this inadvertently positive result. As described above, it may simply be that the playroom is small, and involved the undivided attention of a parent with that child. This might suggest that when hyperactive children are required to sustain their performance to tasks in situations when parents cannot provide them with substantial direction, encouragement, and feedback, the sustained attention of the child cannot be captured by the weaker, intrinsically appealing aspects of the task or by the child's ability to direct and motivate himself.

Clinical Implications

The results of the present studies suggest certain implications for clinical practice with hyperactive children. An important one among these is that the assessment of social interaction conflicts between these children and their parents might offer a more successful way of evaluating precisely those initial difficulties that have brought the parent and child to the clinic. By evaluating the child alone, with the undivided attention of the clinician or examiner, we would not expect a great deal of difficulty from the child. This was in fact the case in a research study by Sleator and Ullmann (1981) in which many hyperactive children did not misbehave in the examining rooms of their pediatricians. Constructing situations in the clinic, or even in the home, that permit the observation of the child's interactions with the actual parents might come close to assessing those interaction conflicts that precipitated the initial referral.

Another implication seems to be that while hyperactive children misbehave in a substantially greater number of situations than their normal peers or siblings, their level of deviant behavior fluctuates quite widely across these different situations. This is contrary to a belief implicit in clinical lore that hyperactive children misbehave everywhere, for if they do not they may not be hyperactive at all. Our research suggests that situational variation is a rather common finding with hyperactive children and should not, by itself, rule out the diagnosis in these children. If clinicians are to better understand the nature of the hyperactive child and his or her deficits, then examining the variation in hyperactive behavior across different settings might be a useful aspect of the initial assessment of such children. While this might be done through direct observation of the child's behavior in various situations, it can also be done through the use of the Home or School Situations Questionnaires (see Barkley, 1981). As many experienced clinicians have learned, knowing what situations seem to provoke misbehavior in children is as important in designing treatment strategies as knowing simply what the behavior problem happens to be.

The results of the drug studies reviewed above indicate that the negative and controlling reactions of the parents to their hyperactive children may, in large measure, simply be responses to the child's deficiencies and difficult behavior rather than being a major cause of it. While this is not to say that parents are completely absolved from any responsibility for the current interaction conflicts in the family, it does suggest that clinicians might refrain from prejudging parental competence simply because significant interaction conflicts are observed with the child. As Bell (1981) suggested, the interaction conflicts may result from the effects of the child on the parent as much as they may reflect parent influences on the child. Clinicians need to accord greater respect for the bidirectionality of effects in family interactions than has previously been the case.

The research reviewed so far offers an interesting glimpse into the manner in which the symptoms of the hyperactive child may precipitate interaction conflicts within the family and how these familial reactions might further exacerbate the child's behavioral problems. Admittedly, this is only a beginning and more research needs to be done, particularly in improving the methodology begun here, so as to further refine our understanding of these interaction problems. Through this refinement might come the promise of developing interventions that are even more specific to the difficulties of the hyperactive child and his or her family than has been the case to date.

REFERENCES

AMERICAN PSYCHIATRIC ASSOCIATION. (1980). *Diagnostic and statistical manual of mental disorders* (3rd ed.). Washington, DC: APA.
BARKLEY, R. A. (1981). *Hyperactive children: A handbook for diagnosis and treatment.* New York: Guilford Press.
BARKLEY, R. A. (1982). Guidelines for defining hyperactivity in children (Attention deficit disorder with hyperactivity). In B. Lahey & A. Kazdin (Eds.), *Advances in clinical child psychology* (Vol. 5). New York: Plenum Press.

BARKLEY, R. A., & CUNNINGHAM, C. E. (1979). The effects of Ritalin on the mother-child interactions of hyperactive children. *Archives of General Psychiatry, 36,* 201-208.

BARKLEY, R. A., & CUNNINGHAM, C. E. (1980). The parent-child interactions of hyperactive children and their modification by stimulant drugs. In R. Knights & D. Bakker (Eds.), *Treatment of hyperactive and learning disordered children.* Baltimore, MD: University Park Press.

BARKLEY, R. A., KARLSSON, J., & POLLARD, S. (in press). Effects of age on the mother-child interactions of ADD-H and normal boys. *Journal of Abnormal Child Psychology.*

BARKLEY, R. A., KARLSSON, J., POLLARD, S., & MURPHY, J. V. (in press). Developmental changes in the mother-child interactions of hyperactive boys: Effects of two dose levels of Ritalin. *Journal of Child Psychology and Psychiatry.*

BARKLEY, R. A., KARLSSON, J., STRZELECKI, E., & MURPHY, J. (1984). Effects of age and Ritalin dosage on the mother-child interactions of hyperactive children. *Journal of Consulting and Clinical Psychology, 52,* 750-758.

BATTLE, E. S., & LACEY, B. (1972). A context for hyperactivity in children over time. *Child Development, 43,* 757-773.

BELL, R. Q. (1968). A reinterpretation of the direction of effects in studies of socialization. *Psychological Review, 75,* 81-95.

BELL, R. Q. (1981). Symposium on parent, child, and reciprocal influences: New experimental approaches. *Journal of Abnormal Child Psychology, 9,* 299-302.

BELL, R. Q., & HARPER, L. (1977). *Child effects on adults.* Hillsdale, NJ: Erlbaum.

CAMPBELL, S. B. (1973). Mother-child interaction in reflective, impulsive, and hyperactive children. *Developmental Psychology, 8,* 341-349.

CAMPBELL, S. B. (1975). Mother-child interaction: A comparison of hyperactive, learning disabled, and normal boys. *American Journal of Orthopsychiatry, 45,* 51-57.

CUNNINGHAM, C. E., & BARKLEY, R. A. (1979). The interactions of hyperactive and normal children with their mothers in free play and structured tasks. *Child Development, 50,* 217-224.

DOUGLAS, V. I. (1972). Stop, look, listen: The problem of sustained attention and impulse control in hyperactive and normal children. *Canadian Journal of Behavioural Science, 4,* 259-282.

DOUGLAS, V. I. (1980). Treatment and training approaches to hyperactivity: Establishing internal or external control. In C. Whalen & B. Henker (Eds.), *Hyperactive children: The social ecology of identification and treatment.* New York: Academic Press.

DOUGLAS, V. I., & PETERS, K. G. (1979). Toward a clearer definition of the attentional deficit of hyperactive children. In G. A. Hale & M. Lewis (Eds.), *Attention and the development of cognitive skills.* New York: Plenum Press.

GOYETTE, C. H., CONNERS, C. K., & ULRICH, R. F. (1978). Normative data on revised Conners Parent and Teacher Rating Scales. *Journal of Abnormal Child Psychology, 6,* 221-236.

LYTTON, H. (1979). Disciplinary encounters between young boys and their mothers and fathers: Is there a contingency system? *Developmental Psychology, 15,* 256-268.

MASH, E., TERDAL, L., & ANDERSON, K. (1973). The Response Class Matrix: A procedure for recording parent-child interactions. *Journal of Consulting and Clinical Psychology, 40,* 163-164.

PATTERSON, G. R. (1976). The aggressive child: Victim and architect of a coercive family system. In E. J. Mash, L. A. Hamerlynck, & L. C. Handy (Eds.), *Behavior modification and families.* New York: Brunner/Mazel.

ROSS, D. M., & ROSS, S. A. (1982). *Hyperactivity: Current issues, research and theory* (2nd ed.). New York: Wiley.

ROUTH, D. K. (1980). Developmental and social aspects of hyperactivity. In C. K. Whalen & B. Henker (Eds.), *Hyperactive children: The social ecology of identification and treatment.* New York: Academic Press.

ROUTH, D. K., & SCHROEDER, C. S. (1976). Standardized playroom observations as indices of hyperactivity. *Journal of Abnormal Child Psychology, 4,* 199-207.

ROUTH, D. K., SCHROEDER, C. S., & O'TUAMA, L. (1974). The development of activity level in children. *Developmental Psychology, 4,* 38-40.

SKINNER, B. F. (1953). *Science and human behavior.* New York: Macmillan.

SLEATOR, E. K., & ULLMANN, R. K. (1981). Can the physician diagnose hyperactivity in the office? *Pediatrics, 67,* 13-17.

WEISS, G., HECHTMAN, L., & PERLMAN, T. (1978). Hyperactives as young adults: School, employers, and self-rating scales obtained during ten-year follow-up evaluation. *American Journal of Orthopsychiatry, 48,* 438-445.

WILLIS, T. J., & LOVAAS, I. (1977). A behavioral approach to treating hyperactive children: The parent's role. In J. G. Millichap (Ed.), *Learning disabilities and related disorders.* Chicago: Yearbook Medical Publications.

11
Parent-Adolescent Conflict: A Developmental Problem of Families

Arthur L. Robin

Adolescence is a period of exponential physiological, cognitive, emotional, and behavioral change. Teenagers are becoming independent of their parents, adjusting to the physical and psychological changes of puberty, developing a sense of identity, establishing strong peer relationships, and preparing for a career and/or vocation (Conger, 1977). The developing adolescent places a great deal of stress upon the family, often resulting in conflict between family members, particularly parents and adolescents.

Parent-adolescent conflict typically takes the form of predominantly verbal arguments between teenagers and their parents concerning specific issues such as curfew, dating, homework, etc. These arguments are characterized by hostile exchanges of accusatory/defensive comments and often do not culminate in a mutually satisfactory resolution of the initial disagreement. The arguments may be sporadic, isolated disagreements or continual, negative interchanges recurring whenever the combatants are in physical proximity. The arguments may spill

The author wishes to acknowledge the contributions of Dr. Sharon Foster, with whom he has collaborated in much of the work described here.

over into the marital arena or may occur despite strong, positive marital bonds.

While parent-adolescent bickering is a ubiquitous developmental phenomenon, under certain circumstances it can intensify to the point where intervention is necessary. In extreme cases, such conflict can propel adolescents toward delinquency, suicide, or psychosomatic disease (Alexander & Parsons, 1982; Conger, 1977; Minuchin, Rosman, & Baker, 1978). How the clinician conceptualizes such negative interactions will influence his or her choice of interventions. One might view parent-adolescent conflict to be a consequence of poor parental management skills, unresolved marital conflict, or organismic deficiencies within individuals, i.e., depression, social skill deficits, etc. Over the past decade we have developed a number of assessment and treatment strategies for coping with parent-teen conflict (Prinz, Foster, Kent, & O'Leary, 1979; Robin, 1980; Robin & Weiss, 1980). Our experiences have led to the formulation of an integrative behavioral-family systems model of parent-adolescent conflict.

The purposes of this chapter are to review the developmental factors promoting parent-adolescent conflict, present a behavioral-family systems account of it, and review an intervention program based upon this model. Research supporting the model and intervention will be briefly summarized.

DEVELOPMENTAL FACTORS AND FAMILY SYSTEMS

Families may be regarded as social systems of members, held together by strong bonds of affection, who exercise mutual control over each others' contingency arrangements (Robin & Foster, 1984). They function as homeostatic systems which self-regulate the behavior of their members within culturally prescribed norms or limits (Jackson, 1965). A family has a definite structure or organization, which permits orderly self-regulation and accomplishment of goals. The individual members also have repertoires of interpersonal problem-solving communication skills and beliefs which both determine and are in part determined by their interactions with other members. Thus, a behavioral-family systems account of parent-adolescent conflict must attend to problem solving, communication skills, belief systems/cognitive sets, the structure of the family, and the function of individuals' behavior within the system.

All of a family's activities take place within a developmental time-

line. As individual members mature, the system evolves in its effort
to maintain homeostatic functioning. Six phases of family development
can be differentiated, each with its own tasks and crises (Carter &
McGoldrick, 1980):

1) between families—the unattached young adult;
2) the newly married couple—the joining of families;
3) the family with young children;
4) the family with adolescents;
5) launching children; and
6) the family in later life.

In the family with adolescents, the primary task is individuation of
the teenager from the parents. The adolescent's striving for independence challenges previously functional interaction patterns, necessitating increased flexibility to permit age-appropriate independence.
Parent-child relationships must shift to permit adolescents increased
decision-making authority and increased opportunity to move easily
in and out of the system. These changes often occur at a time when
parents are past their prime and are preoccupied with their own mid-
life marital and career issues, and foreshadow a shift towards the
parents' concerns for approaching old age. It is, therefore, easy for the
youngster's striving for autonomy to become intertwined with the parents' adjustment to later life.

Simultaneously, the adolescent is developing cognitively. Early adolescence marks the emergence for most youths of formal operational
thought (Inhelder & Piaget, 1958), the ability to reason logically in
ways that younger children do not display. Previously quiescent children now have the ability to present logical arguments to their parents.
Adolescents come increasingly under the control of peer-administered
reinforcement and punishment contingencies, which may conflict with
parental values and contingencies. Given the adolescent's maturing
cognitive abilities, these conflicts set the stage for increased disagreement with parents. Thus, normal adolescent development sets in motion a disruption of homeostatic family relations to which parents must
react.

How the family reacts to disrupted homeostatic functioning deter-
mines the frequency, intensity, and topography of parent-adolescent
conflict. Within a social learning framework, problem-solving communication skills and belief systems are viewed as the "atoms" or
"molecules" of which functional and structural patterns of family in-

teraction are made. When combined in certain proportions to restore homeostatic functioning, they may react explosively to create a full-blown conflict or fuse harmoniously to produce mutually satisfactory relationship outcomes.

PROBLEM SOLVING, COMMUNICATION, AND COGNITION

Research in child development has suggested that democratic problem solving for the resolution of specific parent-teen disputes promotes less conflict and greater achievement of the developmental tasks of adolescence than either authoritarian or permissive conflict resolution techniques (Conger, 1977). Democratic problem solving entails meaningful participation of an adolescent in the decision-making process concerning issues such as curfew or chores, and can be broken down into several stages (D'Zurilla & Goldfried, 1971; Robin & Foster, 1984; Spivack, Platt, & Shure, 1976):

1) *Problem finding*—recognizing the presence of a problem;
2) *Problem definition*—exchanging clear-cut formulations of the problem;
3) *Generation of solutions*—brainstorming creative solutions;
4) *Evaluation*—projecting the benefits and costs of particular solutions;
5) *Decision making*—negotiating a mutually acceptable solution;
6) *Implementation planning*—specifying details for effective solution implementation; and
7) *Verification*—evaluating the effectiveness of solution implementation.

Applying democratic problem solving also requires proficiency in expressive and receptive communication. Parents and teenagers must express opinions assertively but unoffensively, listen to each other attentively, decode each others' messages accurately, and avoid accusations, threats, interruptions, commands, sarcastic remarks, and other negative communication habits. A number of recent studies have confirmed the importance of problem-solving communication skills by demonstrating that clinic-referred distressed families exhibit more negative communication and problem-solving behavior than nondistressed families (Alexander, 1973; Prinz et al., 1979; Prinz, Rosenblum, & O'Leary, 1978; Robin & Weiss, 1980).

When parent-adolescent disagreements arise, the accuracy with which family members process relationship information colors their responses. Beck has identified distorted cognitive styles which are believed to be associated with depression (Beck, 1967, 1976; Beck, Rush, Shaw, & Emery, 1979). Analogous distortions in information processing, which promote intensely angry reactions to parent-teen disagreements, have been identified in families (Robin & Foster, 1984). For example, a parent might engage in absolutistic, dichotomous reasoning, interpreting events in polarized negative or positive categories. A mother who suspects her daughter is sexually active might accuse the girl of being a tramp, whore, or prostitute. Alternatively, family members might display arbitrary inference—the tendency to draw conclusions in the absence of supporting evidence. A father whose son dyes his hair purple and listens to punk-rock music might conclude that the boy is in danger of taking drugs, leading the father to restrict the boys's mobility. Overgeneralization, magnification, and minimization also occur.

A cumulative history of distorted information processing may predispose family members to adhere to rigid, erroneous assumptions about family relations. Common unreasonable beliefs center around themes such as ruination, fairness, obedience/autonomy, and malicious intent:

1) *Ruination.* Parents believe catastrophic consequences will result from adolescents' emission of proscribed behaviors. Teenagers believe parental restrictions will ruin their lives.
2) *Fairness.* Adolescents believe it is a terrible injustice when their parents treat them unfairly or restrict their freedom.
3) *Obedience/autonomy.* Parents expect flawless obedience to parental rules. Adolescents expect complete freedom to do whatever they choose.
4) *Malicious Intent.* Parents believe that teenagers rebel, act out, or misbehave on purpose to hurt their parents.

Inflexible, rigid beliefs translate into rigid positions during disagreements, precluding democratic problem resolution. Distorted information processing predictably elicits negative interpretations of relationship events and hostile affect, interfering with the ability to exercise whatever positive problem-solving communication skills are already in family members' repertoires.

To date, there have not yet been any direct tests of these hypotheses concerning the role of cognitive factors in parent-adolescent conflict. However, research has confirmed the contribution of similar cognitive distortions to marital conflict (Eidelson & Epstein, 1982; Epstein & Eidelson, 1981).

STRUCTURE/FUNCTION

Structure and function are inextricably intertwined. If one views a family's life as a motion picture, a structural analysis entails an examination of the individual frames of the movie while a functional analysis entails an examination of what happens as the frames move through the projector. Families are structured as hierarchical organizations punctuated by differential distribution of power (Haley, 1976; Minuchin, 1974.) Important concepts in a structural analysis are the degree of cohesion, patterns of alignment, coalition, and triangulation within the family (Aponte & VanDeusen, 1981).

The actions of each family member also serve purposes or functions within the system; no one behaves "randomly" within a family. Understanding the purpose of a given action within a particular family requires an analysis of the contingencies which maintain that behavior. The interactions of a family can be depicted behaviorally as interlocking contingency arrangements consisting of sequences of reinforcement, punishment, avoidance, escape, reciprocity, and coercion (Robin & Foster, 1984).

As mentioned earlier, the developmental changes of adolescent independence-seeking challenge existing family structure and functions. Decreasing parental controls can have profound effects on relations between parents and teenagers. As teenagers seek out peer support their relationships with their parents may become less intimate and confiding. Parents who turned to their children for companionship and affection not received from spouses or other adults will no longer have this source of social reinforcement available to them. Those parents whose entire lives were organized around childrearing may find themselves facing a void, and spouses who do not function as a couple except for childrearing will be forced to confront the prospect of a life together without children to preoccupy their interactions. Parents who are accustomed to being in charge at home must now learn to tolerate increased adolescent independence, with the possibility that their offspring may occasionally make unwise decisions which will cause problems. They must become comfortable with their teenagers' increased sexuality, a particularly frightening prospect for many parents.

When parents respond to the disruption of existing homeostatic patterns by resisting or attempting to delay adolescent independence seeking, conflictual interactions escalate. Parents who refuse to grant their youthful offspring increased decision-making power take the risk that the teenagers will either act rebelliously to coerce their parents into granting freedoms or find other ways to punish their parents for authoritarian tactics (i.e., academic failure, delinquency). Parents who attempt to squelch their adolescents' normal heterosexual interests take the risk that their teenagers will act out sexually in an irresponsible fashion. In enmeshed families where parents cannot tolerate the loss of children's affectionate reinforcers, adolescents may appear to remain close to their parents but often develop insidious ways of asserting their autonomy, including the possibility of rebelling by refusing to eat and becoming anorectic (Minuchin et al., 1978).

Closer examination of family systems which resist the striving for autonomy of their youthful members usually reveals that decreased parental control is perceived to be associated with severely aversive consequences for the family and must therefore be avoided, even at the cost of severe parent-child conflict. In some cases, the previously mentioned irrational beliefs about catastrophic outcomes of increased adolescent freedoms motivate parents to restrict their offspring in an overprotective manner. In other cases, the fact that the parents' marriage might disintegrate if the functions served by the dependent behavior of the child are permitted to shift is the overriding factor. Occasionally, an individual parent's self-esteem is so closely tied to the childrearing function that any perceived change in the intensity of the parent-child ties can threaten to elicit severe depressive reaction in the parent.

Since teenagers inevitably seek independence with or without parental encouragement, such problematic family systems are likely to reorganize around the rebellious behavior of the adolescent. When a teenager disobeys rules and regulations, overprotective/authoritarian parents justify further restrictions because their youth's rebellious behavior appears to confirm their dire predictions of the catastrophic consequences of granting autonomy. The cycle of restrictions, rebellion, and negative interactions rapidly becomes self-perpetuating. In marriages threatened by adolescent individuation, the parents unite to discipline a recalcitrant youth, and within a short period of time the rebellious behavior becomes the "glue" binding the couple together.

There remains a great need for empirical investigations of these functional/structural hypotheses concerning parent-adolescent conflict. Although behaviorally oriented clinicians have begun to realize the importance of systemic variables (Foster & Hoier, 1982), they have not yet operationalized and included them in controlled research studies.

ASSESSMENT AND INTERVENTION: OVERVIEW

If parent-adolescent conflict represents a developmental problem in families who are experiencing difficulty reestablishing homeostatic functioning disrupted by adolescent independence seeking, then assessment and intervention should be multifaceted, targeted toward problem-solving communication skills, belief systems, structure, and functions of the families. An intervention program called Problem-Solving Communication Training (PSCT) has been developed which targets these areas (Robin, 1979, 1980; Robin & Foster, 1984). Assessment tools have also been developed to complement this intervention (Prinz et al., 1979; Robin & Weiss, 1980).

The initial assessment phase of PSCT generally lasts between one and one half to three hours and is conducted during one or two sessions. Assessment typically begins with a family interview, followed by administration of several standardized self-report inventories of specific disputes, communication conflict, daily arguments, and marital discord (Prinz et al., 1979). Whenever feasible, an interaction sample is collected by audiotaping the family discussing a dispute and later coding the audiotape with either a global-inferential (Prinz & Kent, 1978) or detailed frequency-based coding system (Robin & Weiss, 1980). Formal assessment concludes with the development of a therapeutic contract specifying goals for change, treatment procedures, responsibilities of the clients, and responsibilities of the therapist. The present discussion will emphasize treatment rather than assessment. More detailed discussion of assessment can be found elsewhere (Robin, 1980; Robin & Foster, 1984).

Problem-solving communication training combines problem solving, communication skill training, cognitive restructuring, and the selected use of family systems techniques necessary to change structure and function. The therapist blends these components into a comprehensive behavioral family therapy geared to the presenting problems and interaction patterns of the family.

Each family participates in seven to 15 one-hour treatment sessions. Following completion of the initial assessment, problem solving is usually the first component to be introduced. Early sessions are organized primarily around the issues to be resolved, with one issue addressed per session. During the first session, the therapist uses instructions, modeling, behavior rehearsal, and corrective feedback to guide the family through the stages of problem solving (described below) for a mild-to-moderate intensity dispute. Afterwards, the family is sent home to implement the solution.

At successive sessions, increasingly severe disputes are problem-solved, or previously agreed upon solutions which failed are renegotiated. During problem-solving training, negative communication habits which interfere with productive verbal interchanges are targeted for change. Beginning with the second session, the therapist uses correction, modeling, behavior rehearsal, and feedback to change one or two communication targets at a time.

By the third or fourth session, family members' absolutistic beliefs and distorted information-processing styles become evident, often in the form of resistance to compromise or negotiation. Verbal disputation, exaggeration and humor, and reframing techniques are used to clarify and challenge unreasonable cognitions, and both parents and adolescent are asked to conduct "experiments" to disconfirm absolutistic beliefs.

To program generalization across time and settings, the therapist assigns homework, including implementation of solutions, additional discussions of disputes to be held at home, and tasks incorporating newly acquired skills/attitudes into daily living. Time is allotted at the beginning and end of each session for discussion of homework assignments.

Throughout all of the treatment sessions the therapist attends to structural and functional interaction patterns, generating hypotheses about interlocking contingency arrangements, cohesion, coalitions, and triangulation. In the later sessions, when the family has acquired basic problem-solving communication skills, session format is more flexible. Instead of organizing sessions around specific disputes or negative communication habits, the therapist plans strategies to address structural/functional problems. If marital conflict and/or individual organismic difficulties are problems, one or more individual or couple sessions might then be conducted.

Termination is approached by gradually increasing the interval between sessions. By termination, a successfully treated family will have acquired skills and beliefs which will permit continued resolution of disputes in the future and will also have resolved many of their presenting problems.

More details will now be given concerning components of PSCT.

PROBLEM SOLVING

Families are taught a four-step outline of problem solving, which represents a telescoped version of the seven components of democratic problem solving outlined earlier in the chapter: problem definition, generation of alternatives, decision making, and planning solution implementation. A fifth step, renegotiation, is invoked when the family fails to resolve a dispute through implementing an initial solution. In keeping with the developmental emphasis on upgrading the adolescent's position within the power hierarchy of the family, the therapist strongly encourages equal participation of parents and adolescents in problem solving by treating the adolescent's opinions respectfully, blocking parental monopolization of the conversation, and stopping parental discounting of the youth's opinions.

During the problem definition phase of the discussion, each member is asked to express clearly his or her perspective concerning the topic under consideration, and the others are asked to reflect back to the speaker their understanding of his or her definition. An adequate problem definition statement is concise, nonaccusatory, and addresses behaviors, feelings, and situations, not personality characteristics. An adequate reflection restates the listener's perceptions of the speaker's point accurately, without deletions or additions. Inadequate statements are corrected, with participants being asked to rephrase their statements several times if necessary.

During the generation of alternative solutions phase of the discussion, each member takes turns listing all of their ideas as to possible solutions to the problem. The therapist prompts them to generate creative, outrageous ideas but to refrain from evaluating them. One member is assigned the task of recording the ideas in writing. The therapist may suggest additional ideas if the members "run dry."

When the family has generated eight to ten ideas, several of which go beyond their initial positions, the therapist teaches them to decide upon an acceptable idea by projecting the consequences of implementing each idea, rating it positively or negatively (recorded in writing), and agreeing to implement the one or more ideas rated positively by everyone. If the family fails to reach a consensus, the therapist directively guides them to negotiate a compromise by brainstorming and evaluating all of the possible compromises, then bargaining with each other. Strategies for overcoming resistance to negotiation using social-psychological/attributional techniques have been detailed elsewhere (Robin, 1981). The use of cognitive restructuring for this purpose will be discussed later in the chapter.

The fourth phase of problem solving, implementation planning, consists of specifying the details which are necessary to put an agreed upon solution into practice. It is decided who will do what, when, where, and in what way. An oral and/or written procedure is designed to monitor solution compliance. Then the family is sent home to implement the solution.

At the beginning of the next session, the therapist requests a report of the implementation. If the solution worked, the family is praised, and the therapist moves ahead to a new issue. However, if implementation was not successful, the therapist reframes the failure within a constructive, nonaccusatory framework and helps the family to renegotiate another solution.

COMMUNICATION TRAINING

Based upon assessment information and observations of in-session interactions, the therapist assembles a list of problematic communication patterns for each family. Common negative communication targets include talking through a third person, accusing, putting down, interrupting, lecturing, moralizing, talking sarcastically, failing to make eye contact, fidgeting, mindreading, getting off the topic, dwelling on the past, and commanding. Alternative, positive communication behaviors include talking directly to another person, making I-statements, accepting responsibility, listening without interrupting, making brief non-preaching remarks, talking in a neutral tone of voice, establishing eye contact when interacting with another, sitting in a relaxed fashion, paraphrasing, sticking to the topic, sticking to the present and future, and suggesting ideas in a non-imperative manner.

One or two targets are selected for change during each session. The therapist describes the negative response, models an alternative positive response, and prepares the family for correction. Whenever the inappropriate response is emitted, the therapist interrupts the discussion, labels the behavior, prompts and/or models a positive response, and requires the family to "replay the scene." Over time, the therapist modifies a variety of negative communication patterns through the use of feedback, instructions, modeling, and behavior rehearsal. Eventually, parents and adolescents are assigned the task of self-monitoring and correcting their own negative communication habits. Readers interested in further information concerning communication training might consult a number of sources (Alexander & Parsons, 1982; Gottman, Notarius, Gonso, & Markman, 1976; Guerney, 1977; Jacobson & Margolin, 1979; Robin, 1980).

COGNITIVE RESTRUCTURING

Strategies for cognitive restructuring are derived from Ellis' rational-emotive therapy (Ellis & Grieger, 1977) and Beck's cognitive therapy (Beck et al., 1979). The therapist follows five general steps: 1) identify the inappropriate cognition; 2) challenge it; 3) model a more appropriate alternative; 4) propose an experiment designed to test the validity of the belief; and 5) help the family plan to complete the experiment at home.

In some cases, family members clearly identify their own unreasonable beliefs, as when a compulsive father asserts that children who fail to clean up their rooms grow up to be irresponsible adults, or an overprotective mother tearfully reveals her anxieties that her daughter will take drugs and have sex if she is permitted to date before the age of 18. In other cases, in-session behavior cues the therapist to probe for rigid cognitions, as when negotiations repeatedly break down during problem solving. The therapist makes liberal use of humor, exaggeration, and Socratic reasoning in an unoffensive manner to make the family aware of the unreasonableness of their beliefs.

Distorted cognitions can be challenged by exaggerating them to absurd proportions and dissecting their consequences with a sharp but smooth cutting edge. The therapist might, for example, point out to the father who believes the teenager's failure to clean his room will lead to irresponsible adult behavior that, since most teenagers occasionally fail to clean their rooms, this belief implies that most adults are irresponsible. Furthermore, the father can probably recall at least one occasion during his own adolescent years when he failed to clean his room, and he certainly does not consider himself an irresponsible adult. Pursuing this line of reasoning doggedly but politely usually helps to challenge unreasonable beliefs. The therapist may also request the parents and adolescent to marshall the evidence in support of and in opposition to the veracity of a particular belief, and permit the client's inability to make a convincing argument to serve as the basis for the challenge. In any event, caustic confrontations backfire and are to be avoided.

To model realistic, flexible thought processes, the therapist suggests transforming extremist modifiers such as "should," "must," and "always" into more tentative modifiers such as "it would be nice if," "I would be pleased if," and "as often as possible." Emphasis is placed upon logical deductions and evidence-based conclusions instead of arbitrary, overgeneralized reasoning. For example, the belief that "children who fail to clean their rooms grow up to be irresponsible adults" might be altered to "children who fail to clean their rooms have sloppy rooms which annoy their parents, but no one has proved such behavior leads to adult irresponsibility."

Next, the therapist suggests an "experiment" to test the veracity of alternative cognitions in order that family members convince themselves, based upon their personal experiences rather than external persuasion, of the utility of adopting more flexible cognitive sets. A helpful experiment consists of a task to be completed at home, with clearly specified outcomes which confirm or disconfirm the beliefs. Possibilities include: 1) implementing a solution on a trial basis and determining whether the dire consequences predicted to follow do in fact transpire; 2) surveying other families to determine whether their experiences confirm the belief; 3) reading a book or collecting other published data concerning the belief; or 4) observing family members' behavior to see whether they act in accordance with predictions based upon the belief.

Finally, an agreement is reached concerning who will do what, when, and how to conduct the experiment. Of course, the amount of time devoted to cognitive restructuring will depend upon the presenting problems of each family. In some cases, cognitive restructuring may be used on a "catch-it-correct-it" basis throughout a session; in other cases, the therapist may devote several entire sessions (usually later in treatment) to unreasonable beliefs.

STRUCTURE AND FUNCTIONS

A coordinated strategy is developed to address structural and functional aspects of parent-adolescent conflict based upon assessment information and the therapist's impressions derived from the first few treatment sessions. The therapist formulates a hypothesis about a particular interlocking contingency arrangement in need of change, identifies a more desirable contingency arrangement, and then assigns tasks to be completed within the sessions and at home designed to bring about the desired change. Often, the other components of treatment (problem solving, communication training, cognitive restructuring) serve as vehicles for creating tasks to change structure and/or functions. Examples of such interventions will be given here, although an exhaustive review is not possible.

One common problem arises when adolescents become inappropriately involved in their parents' marital affairs. A mother and father who disagree about a variety of marital and childrearing issues may engage in many heated arguments with an implicit or explicit threat of separation and divorce. The arguments and threat of separation are aversive to the adolescent, who over time may learn to emit an escalating chain of rebellious behaviors to coerce the parents to cease marital fights by refocusing their attention on teenage misbehavior. The following sequence of events often repeats:

1) the parents have a marital fight;
2) the youth misbehaves;
3) the parents stop their fight to discipline the youth;
4) the youth ceases misbehaving;
5) the parents cease attending to a now well-behaved youth;
6) marital fights resume; and
7) adolescent misbehavior resumes.

A behavioral analysis of this sequence depicts the functional interdependence between the parents' and teenager's behavior in terms of interlocking three-term contingency arrangements. For example, if marital fights are aversive to the adolescent and the teenager's misbehavior reliably results in cessation of a marital fight, then the cessation of marital arguments is functioning as a negative reinforcer for adolescent misbehavior. If marital fights are also unpleasant for the parents and their adolescent's misbehavior coerces them to terminate fighting and discipline the youth, then adolescent misbehavior is helping the parents avoid protracted arguments, and can be viewed as serving an avoidance function in the parents' marriage with respect to fighting. Thus, the self-perpetuating sequence of interactions serves a function for each family member. In systems terms, the adolescent's misbehavior may be the "glue" which binds the parents together. The topography of such adolescent misbehavior varies widely but often includes academic failure, truancy, shoplifting, and alcohol or drug-related problems.

The therapist's goal is to remove the adolescent from the marital struggle and help the parents resolve marital issues directly. Then, the adolescent will no longer need to act out to stop parental fights and save the marriage. Parent-teen disputes can also be settled directly. In some cases, the therapist can give a family feedback that marital discord is interfering with resolution of parent-teen conflict and invite the couple to attend marital therapy concurrently with family sessions.

Often, couples seeking treatment for child problems resist acknowledging marital discord, and a more subtle approach is necessary. The therapist might select a parent-adolescent issue to problem solve which is likely to be tied to the interlocking negative reinforcement contingency arrangement. The family might then be asked to describe the sequence of events surrounding the parent-adolescent dispute. As the family describes this sequence, the therapist can point out how parent-adolescent conflict consistently follows marital disagreements and reframe the adolescent's misbehavior as an attempt to "help" the parents deal with their own problems. By asking the adolescent to express his or her perceptions of the parents' marriage, as well as his or her cognitive, emotional, and behavioral responses to their arguments, the therapist can highlight the interlocking contingency arrangement and in a timely fashion give the couple the option of participating in marital therapy.

A variation of the theme of inappropriate adolescent involvement in marital affairs occurs when the parents fight with each other through their adolescent. Each parent attempts to persuade the adolescent to take his or her side against the other, and the adolescent vacillates between supporting mother or father. Family systems therapists call this sequence of contingencies "triangulation" (Aponte & VanDeusen, 1981). A father may undermine a mother's attempt to discipline an adolescent, promoting mother-son arguments and "punishing" his wife for some past behavior she directed toward him; a mother may act the same way toward her husband and son. An adolescent typically takes advantage of this type of parental discord to break rules and avoid punishments. The therapist can change triangulated interactions by first requiring the parents to negotiate joint ground rules for disciplining the adolescent, and then requiring the parents to problem solve issues with the adolescent. Homework can be assigned which requires the parents to check with each other before responding to adolescent misbehavior. If the parents are unable to agree upon a joint approach for dealing with their adolescent, the therapist can then point out the need for marital sessions.

A second common functional/structural problem arises in highly enmeshed families where parents resist adolescent independence seeking, possibly because of the loss of affectionate reinforcement that might occur when the adolescent spends increased time away from home, or possibly because of unrealistic cognitions about how family members should behave. To alter these patterns, the therapist can target in-session interactions which exemplify enmeshment. Common targets include interrupting, mindreading, and talking for another member. These behaviors can be corrected through the use of feedback, instructions, and behavior rehearsal.

In addition, the therapist can select topics for problem solving which represent privacy issues (adolescent selecting own clothing, being alone in his or her room, keeping secrets, etc.). Tasks designed to disengage family members can be assigned as homework. These might include the adolescent's staying for a weekend at a friend's house, the adolescent going to camp for a summer, or one family member keeping secrets from another. Cognitive restructuring can correct such myths as "I'm a bad parent if my son doesn't always confide in me," or "It's disloyal to my parents to spend time with my friends."

Readers interested in additional discussion of interventions for altering family structure and function might consult the family systems literature (Alexander & Parsons, 1982; Haley, 1976, 1980; Madanes, 1981; Minuchin, 1974).

EFFECTIVENESS OF PROBLEM-SOLVING COMMUNICATION TRAINING

Three outcome studies have been conducted to evaluate the effectiveness of Problem-Solving Communication Training (PSCT). A brief overview of these studies will be given here.

In an initial investigation of whether a basic problem-solving communication training package was more effective than no treatment for reducing mother-adolescent conflict, 22 self-referred mother-adolescent dyads were randomly assigned to either five sessions of PSCT or a wait-list control (Robin et al., 1977). Treatment was restricted to the skill training component of the intervention without emphasis on cognitive, structural, or functional variables.

Measures were administered before and after treatment or the wait-list period, and included audiotaped discussions of conflictual issues coded for the frequency of problem-solving communication behavior and questionnaires of perceived communication and conflict at home. Treated dyads made significant gains on problem-solving communication behavior; control dyads did not. Analyses of questionnaire measures revealed no significant gains for treated dyads compared to control dyads. This preliminary study indicated that treatment was associated with the acquisition of skills but not the reduction of conflict at home.

In a second study, Foster, Prinz, and O'Leary (1983) broadened the intervention to include homework assignments designed to enhance generalization of basic skills to the home environment and examined the maintenance of treatment effects over time. Twenty-eight families (dyads and triads) were randomly assigned to either a wait-list control or seven sessions of one of two treatments. One treatment emphasized problem-solving communication skill-building, with no discussion of skill use at home, and the other combined skill-building and skill use at home. Assignments were given to practice the use of problem-solving communication skills at home, and session time was devoted to discussion of home applications.

Measures were administered before and after treatment, and six to eight weeks after completion of treatment. Measures included audiotaped discussions coded for the frequency of positive and negative problem-solving communication behaviors and questionnaires tapping levels of specific disputes, daily arguments, communication-conflict behavior, and goal attainment. It should be noted that Foster et al. (1983) employed previously validated measures while Robin et al. (1977) did not.

Treated families displayed minimal gains on problem-solving communication behavior, in contrast to the findings of Robin et al. (1977). However, analyses of questionnaire measures revealed significant gains for treated families compared to controls on goal attainment, specific disputes, and communication-conflict behavior. There were no differences between the skill training alone and the skill training plus generalization programming conditions at post-assessment.

While most treatment gains were maintained at follow-up, a small number of measures showed continued improvement for the skill training group but some deterioration for the generalization group. Contrary to predictions, generalization strategies appeared to impede maintenance of at least selected gains.

A third investigation compared PSCT to a best-alternative treatment group as well as a wait-list condition (Robin, 1981). Thirty-three families (dyads and triads) were randomly assigned to a wait-list condition or seven sessions of one of two treatments. The PSCT condition blended skill training, generalization programming, and cognitive restructuring. The best-alternative treatment condition was a melange of family systems, eclectic, or psychodynamic family therapy included to provide realistic, ethically sound "controls" for placebo and therapist factors.

Measures similar to those employed by Foster et al. (1983) were administered before treatment, after treatment, and at eight to ten week follow-up intervals following completion of treatment. Treated parents and adolescents improved significantly more than the wait-list group on questionnaire measures of specific disputes and perceived communication-conflict at home as well as coded audiotapes of problem-solving communication behavior. PSCT improved more than the best-alternative treatment group on problem-solving communication behavior, but the two groups showed similar gains on questionnaire measures. Treatment gains were maintained at follow-up, but only 60% of the original sample completed the follow-up measures, suggesting caution in interpreting these data.

Despite their differences and individual methodological shortcomings, these three studies taken together do suggest that PSCT can ameliorate perceived conflict and specific disputes at home and lead to the acquisition of positive problem-solving communication behavior. Positive changes were maintained over short follow-up intervals, and were obtained with mother-adolescent dyads as well as mother-father-adolescent triads.

The discrepancies between the results of the three studies also make it clear that much remains to be learned about the conditions under which PSCT is an effective, appropriate intervention for the developmental conflicts of parents and adolescents. Considerable variability was evident in the amount of improvement across families and studies, and several important questions were not at all addressed, including long-term maintenance of treatment gains and the importance of functional/structural interventions.

CONCLUSION

Research and clinical experiences with PSCT and a behavioral-family systems model have raised as many questions as they have answered. In summary, I wish to consider critical issues for future investigation.

What types of families benefit most from which components of the intervention? Clinical experiences have suggested that skill training plus cognitive restructuring is sufficient to produce lasting change in families where the onset of conflict is a recent phenomenon and overprotective/authoritarian parents are reacting to the exaggerated rebelliousness of young adolescents. However, additional interventions appear necessary for severely distressed families characterized by an onset of parent-child conflict prior to adolescence, marital discord, extreme enmeshment, cross-generational alliances, and/or chronic triangulation. Large-scale factorial investigations examining treatment components by family-type interactions would be desirable to test these hypotheses and determine the contribution of each component to PSCT. Of course, it is recognized that such investigations are extremely difficult to conduct, and require a great deal of time, manpower, and financial resources. Alternatively, investigators might include measures of family characteristics in smaller scale outcome studies. I have begun to include measures of family cohesion and adaptability in my own ongoing outcome research. By correlating such measures with therapeutic outcome, we can begin to learn which types of families respond best to which types of treatment components.

What therapist characteristics and therapist behaviors are associated with positive outcomes using PSCT? Barton and Alexander (1981) noted that a combination of relationship and structuring skills are necessary to achieve positive outcomes with an intervention similar to PSCT. What is the appropriate balance of structure and flexibility for a therapist to maintain during a problem-solving training discussion? While the therapist must remain flexible enough to deviate from a preplanned agenda in response to a crisis, repeated deviations to explore interesting material can lead to a chaotic outcome. How do variables such as the therapist's age, sex, marital status, childrearing experiences, and own family-of-origin experiences influence reactions to particular parent-adolescent interactions? How can the therapist best respond to difficulties engaging resistant family members in treatment and maintain their cooperation? At the present time, there is much practical advice available to interested therapists (Gurman, 1981), but little empirical data to support particular modes of therapeutic response to these problems.

The behavioral-family systems model of parent-adolescent conflict presented here is also largely untested, with the exception of several studies concerning problem-solving communication deficits in distressed and nondistressed families (Alexander, 1973; Robin & Weiss, 1980). The practical limitations of adopting either a purely behavioral or a purely family systems approach to treatment have led to the present attempt to integrate these two frameworks, but much work remains to be done before a clear-cut, logically consistent model of parent-adolescent conflict will emerge. How, for example, can concepts such as "homeostasis," "enmeshment," or "triangulation" be clearly depicted with behavioral operations?

Correlational and longitudinal investigations are needed to test specific behavioral-family systems hypotheses. Does adolescent independence-seeking indeed disrupt family homeostasis, or are other factors responsible for the onset of parent-adolescent conflict? Is there a core set of distorted beliefs common to families in conflict, or are such distortions idiosyncratic to particular families? How do skill deficits, cognitive distortions, and structural/functional problems interact to produce conflict? Is a behavioral-family systems model a post-hoc exercise in semantic reductionism or does it contribute in a meaningful manner to the development of new assessment tools and treatment programs?

At the present time in the history of child and family behavior therapy, there has been a great deal of movement toward an integration with developmental psychology and family systems approaches (Alexander & Parsons, 1982; Birchler & Spinks, 1980; Foster & Hoier, 1982). The treatment program and theoretical model outlined here represents one such endeavor. Only through continued emphasis on the empirical tradition of behavior therapy will such attempts ultimately prove fruitful.

REFERENCES

ALEXANDER, J. F. (1973). Defensive and supportive communications in normal and deviant families. *Journal of Consulting and Clinical Psychology, 40,* 223-231.
ALEXANDER, J., & PARSONS, B. V. (1982). *Functional family therapy.* Monterey, CA: Brooks/Cole.
APONTE, H. J., & VANDEUSEN, J. M. (1981). Structural family therapy. In A. S. Gurman & D. P. Kniskern (Eds.), *Handbook of family therapy.* New York: Brunner/Mazel.
BARTON, C., & ALEXANDER, J. F. (1981). Functional family therapy. In A. S. Gurman & D. P. Kniskern (Eds.), *Handbook of family therapy.* New York: Brunner/Mazel.
BECK, A. T. (1967). *Depression: Clinical, experimental, and theoretical aspects.* New York: Hoeber.
BECK, A. T. (1976). *Cognitive therapy and the emotional disorders.* New York: International Universities Press.
BECK, A. T., RUSH, A. J., SHAW, B. F., & EMERY, G. (1979). *Cognitive therapy of depression.* New York: Guilford Press.
BIRCHLER, G. R., & SPINKS, S. H. (1980). Behavioral-systems marital and family therapy: Integration and clinical application. *The American Journal of Family Therapy, 8,* 6-28.

CARTER, E. A., & McGOLDRICK, M. (Eds.). (1980). *The family life cycle: A framework for family therapy.* New York: Gardner Press.

CONGER, J. J. (1977). *Adolescence and youth: Psychological development in a changing world* (2nd ed.). New York: Harper & Row.

D'ZURILLA, T. J., & GOLDFRIED, M. R. (1971). Problem solving and behavior modification. *Journal of Abnormal Psychology, 78,* 197-226.

EIDELSON, R. J., & EPSTEIN, N. (1982). Cognition and relationship maladjustment: Development of a measure of dysfunctional relationship beliefs. *Journal of Consulting and Clinical Psychology, 50,* 715-720.

ELLIS, A., & GRIEGER, R. (1977). *Handbook of rational emotive therapy.* New York: Springer-Verlag.

EPSTEIN, N., & EIDELSON, R. J. (1981). Unrealistic beliefs of clinical couples: Their relationship to expectations, goals, and satisfaction. *The American Journal of Family Therapy, 9,* 13-22.

FOSTER, S. L., & HOIER, T. (1982). Behavioral and systems family therapies: A comparison of theoretical assumptions. *The American Journal of Family Therapy, 10,* 13-23.

FOSTER, S. L., PRINZ, R. J., & O'LEARY, K. D. (1983). Impact of problem-solving communication training and generalization programming procedures on family conflict. *Child and Family Behavior Therapy, 5,* 1-23.

GOTTMAN, J., NOTARIUS, C., GONSO, J., & MARKMAN, H. (1976). *A couple's guide to communication.* Champaign, IL: Research Press.

GUERNEY, B. G. (1977). *Relationship enchancement.* San Francisco: Jossey-Bass.

GURMAN, A. S. (Ed.). (1981). *Questions and answers in the practice of family therapy.* New York: Brunner/Mazel.

HALEY, J. (1976). *Problem-solving therapy.* San Francisco: Jossey-Bass.

HALEY, J. (1980). *Leaving home: The therapy of disturbed young people.* New York: McGraw-Hill.

INHELDER, B., & PIAGET, J. (1958). *The growth of logical thinking from childhood to adolescence.* New York: Basic Books.

JACKSON, D. D. (1965). The study of the family. *Family Process, 4,* 1-20.

JACOBSON, N. S., & MARGOLIN, G. (1979). *Marital therapy: Strategies based on social learning and behavior exchange principles.* New York: Brunner/Mazel.

MADANES, C. (1981). *Strategic family therapy.* San Francisco: Jossey-Bass.

MINUCHIN, S. (1974). *Families and family therapy.* Cambridge, MA: Harvard University Press.

MINUCHIN, S., ROSMAN, B., & BAKER, L. (1978). *Psychosomatic families.* Cambridge, MA: Harvard University Press.

PRINZ, R. J., FOSTER, S., KENT, R. N., & O'LEARY, K. D. (1979). Multivariate assessment of conflict in distressed and nondistressed mother-adolescent dyads. *Journal of Applied Behavior Analysis, 12,* 691-700.

PRINZ, R. N., & KENT, R. (1978). Recording parent-adolescent interactions without the use of frequency or interval-by-interval coding. *Behavior Therapy, 9,* 602-604.

PRINZ, R. J., ROSENBLUM, R. S., & O'LEARY, K. D. (1978). Affective communication differences between distressed and nondistressed mother-adolescent dyads. *Journal of Abnormal Child Psychology, 6,* 373-383.

ROBIN, A. L. (1979). Problem-solving communication training: A behavioral approach to the treatment of parent-adolescent conflict. *The American Journal of Family Therapy, 7,* 69-82.

ROBIN, A. L. (1980). Parent-adolescent conflict: A skill training approach. In D. P. Rathjen & J. P. Foreyt (Eds.), *Social competence: Interventions for children and adults.* New York: Pergamon Press.

ROBIN, A. L. (1981). A controlled evaluation of problem-solving communication training with parent-adolescent conflict. *Behavior Therapy, 12,* 593-609.

ROBIN, A. L., & FOSTER, S. L. (1984). Problem-solving communication training: A behavioral-family systems approach to parent-adolescent conflict. In P. Karoly & J. Steffen (Eds.), *Adolescent behavior disorders: Foundations and contemporary concerns*. Lexington, MA: D. C. Heath.

ROBIN, A. L., KENT, R., O'LEARY, K. D., FOSTER, S., & PRINZ, R. (1977). An approach to teaching parents and adolescents problem-solving communication skills: A preliminary report. *Behavior Therapy, 8*, 639-643.

ROBIN, A. L., & WEISS, J. G. (1980). Criterion-related validity of behavioral and self-report measures of problem-solving communication skills in distressed and non-distressed parent-adolescent dyads. *Behavioral Assessment, 2*, 339-352.

SPIVACK, G., PLATT, J. J., & SHURE, M. B. (1976). *The problem-solving approach to adjustment*. San Francisco: Jossey-Bass.

Name Index

Subject Index